INTERMITTENT FASTING FOR WOMEN OVER 50

THE ESENTIAL GUIDE TO WEIGHT LOSS

Table of content

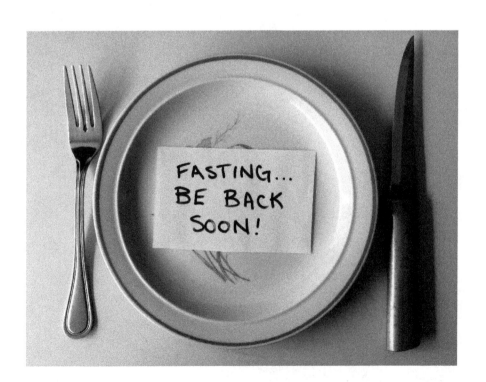

INTRODUCTION

For almost as long as mankind, people have fasted. Now and again, this was a result of the need on the grounds that no food was accessible.

In different cases, it was accomplished for strict reasons. Numerous religions, for example, Christianity, Buddhism, and Islam, order types of fasting.

In nature, the two people and creatures normally fast on the off chance that they are debilitated.

Fasting is normal, as our bodies are intended to deal with broadened periods without eating.

At the point when you fast, your body experiences a few unique procedures and changes, which include an assortment of variables, for example, hormones and qualities, which add to cell fix forms.

While numerous individuals fast to shed pounds and proficiently limit their calories to drive their bodies to consume progressively fat, others fast to diminish glucose and insulin levels. Furthermore, fasting likewise expands the Human Growth Hormone (HGH). Different examinations show that intermittent fasting may secure against various types of infections, for example, type II diabetes, coronary illness, malignant growth, and Alzheimer's sickness, to give some examples.

There are three fundamental types of intermittent fasting.

1. The 16/8 Method – We fastly addressed this one. It includes fasting for 16 hours every day and just eating among early afternoon and 8:00 PM. In any case, you can without much of a stretch modify this window to oblige your life's calendar better. Simply make a point to fast for 16 hours in a row.

2. The 5:2 Diet – This includes eating typically consistently, with the exception of two days of every week limiting caloric admission to 500 to 600 calories.

3. Eat-Stop-Eat – This fast requires a few times per week not having anything from dinner one day until dinner the next day, which is basically a 24-hour fast.

Ways which intermittent works

Since the body works diversely when it's in "feast" versus "starvation" mode, fasting might be helpful for weight loss.

Subsequent to eating a feast, the body takes a few hours to process the food, while burning what it just expended. At the point when you consistently fuel your body, it consumes that fuel rather than your fat fuel holds. This is particularly valid in the event that you devour considerable characteristics of starches or sugars, as your body will normally consume this as a wellspring of vitality over putting away fat.

At the point when your body is fasting, your body doesn't pull from its ongoing food saves for vitality, which implies that it depends on your fat stockpiling. It will, at that point, pull from this stockpiling for vitality to fuel your body.

The equivalent is genuine when you exercise while fasting. On the off chance that the body doesn't have a promptly accessible stockpile of glucose and glycogen to pull from, it draws from the fat put away in your cells.

Since our bodies respond to eating food by creating insulin, when your body isn't constantly overwhelmed with a lot of this hormone, it's bound to devour it effectively. The body is generally touchy to this hormone subsequent to fasting. By changing the measure of insulin generation, you can hypothetically improve your body's affectability to insulin, which can assist you with shedding pounds and manufacture more muscle.

In case you're keen on investigating Intermittent fasting, however, aren't sure if it's appropriate for you, consider this key focuses.

- **Meet Your Goals** – Not all calories are equivalent, and caloric limitation assumes a noteworthy job in getting more fit. At the point when individuals fast, it makes it simpler for them to limit their general caloric admission through the span of a day or week.

- **Simplify Your Day** – Instead of planning up to six little dinners daily, by avoiding a couple of, individuals can spare important time settling on fewer choices, doing less shopping, and eating out.

- **Better Hormones** – Intermittent fasting can help advance more grounded insulin affectability while expanding the development hormone, the two of which are fundamental segments for weight loss and muscle gain.

- **Boost Your Brain** – There are numerous Ted discusses how fasting can help check conditions, for example, dementia, Alzheimer's, and Parkinson's.

As usual, before leaving on a weight loss venture, it is ideal to counsel with a restorative expert initially.

HISTORY OF INTERMITTENT FASTING

Contrasted with customary "dieting," fasting is straightforward and unambiguous. It's constantly been finished. You, as of now, unwittingly do IF at whatever point you skip breakfast or dinner. Generally, during tracker gatherer days, our predecessors were in a fasting state while looking for food. At the point when agribusiness was set up, human advancement came straightaway. Be that as it may, when food was rare or seasons changed, fasting was as yet a lifestyle. Urban communities and manors put away grain and restored meat for the Page 3 winter. Prior to the water system, absence of downpour implied starvation, and individuals fasted to make they put away food keep going to the extent that this would be possible until the downpours returned and it was workable for harvests to endure once more. Religions thrived right now individuals living nearer together, sharing and spreading conviction and customs. What's more, religions additionally endorsed fasting. Hinduism calls fasting "Vaasa" and watches it during uncommon days or celebrations, as individual compensation, or to respect their own divine beings. Islam and Judaism have Ramadan and Yom Kippur, when it's illegal to work, eat, drink, wash, wear cowhide, and engage in sexual relations. In Catholicism, it's a month and a half of fasting before Easter or before Holy Week.

Nonetheless, fasting would grow past a basic endurance system as individuals started creating strict convictions. Pretty much every significant religion incorporates a few examples of fasting. For instance, Catholicism incorporates fasting practices during the festival of Lent.

These activities incorporate constraining their admission of meat and, in any case limiting their calories.

In Buddhism, adherents fast to help purge the brain and discharge the body from a requirement for customary food. The thought behind this conduct is to control the body's contrary inclinations and increment an individual's inward otherworldly quality. Some of the time, Buddhists had the option to transform their capacity to fastly into an unimaginable force. For instance, think about how Gandhi had the option to pick up autonomy for India just by driving his kin with hunger strikes.

This data shows that fasting is a long way from abnormal conduct or something that is perilous or unsuitable to the body. Actually, intermittent fasting is something that can have numerous benefits for an individual on the off chance that it is taken care of appropriately.

Before examining these benefits and why they happen, it merits understanding a couple of people who have attempted intermittent fasting previously.

The cutting edge time of horticulture and manufacturing plant loaded "food" (or food-like substances) has totally changed the manner in which people see and expend food every day, prompting the clothing rundown of medical issues that our general public faces today. Despite the fact that IF is an old practice, the science behind its numerous medical advantages is simply as of late being presented to standard society. At the point when you fast, you essentially permit your body to normally wash down, fix and recover itself for ideal capacity. Three of the principle wellbeing advancing components related to fasting incorporate the metabolic guideline of circadian science, the gut microbiome, and diverse way of life practices. Circadian Biology Humans (and different life forms) have advanced to build up a circadian clock that guarantees physiological procedures inside your body are performed at ideal occasions for the duration of the day. These circadian rhythms happen across 24-hour light-dim cycles and impact changes in science and conduct. Interfering with this circadian beat contrarily impacts metabolism, which adds to stoutness and related sicknesses, for example, type 2 diabetes, cardiovascular malady, and malignant growth. This is the place intermittent fasting comes in. Sustaining signals appear to be the principle timing prompt for how your circadian rhythms capacity and, in this way, control certain metabolic, physiological, and social pathways that add to by and large wellbeing and life span. Certain social intercessions, for example, (you got it!) intermittent fasting can help synchronize your circadian rhythms prompting improved vacillations in quality articulation, reconstructing of vitality metabolism, and improved hormonal and bodyweight guideline, all factors that assume an imperative job in upgrading your wellbeing results. The Gut Microbiome The gastrointestinal (GI) tract, otherwise called the "gut," assumes a critical job in managing a few procedures inside your body. Page 5 Many functions of the gut (and almost every physiological and biochemical capacity in your body) are affected by your circadian musicality portrayed above. For instance, gastric discharging, bloodstream, and metabolic reactions to glucose are more prominent during the daytime than around evening time. Thus, almost certainly, a constantly upset circadian cadence can influence gut work, adding to hindered metabolism and expanded hazard for incessant ailment. The gut microbiome, otherwise called our "second brain," has been the subject of broad research in both wellbeing and sickness because of its significant association in human metabolism, physiology, nutrition, and resistant capacity

MEANING AND AUTOPHAGY OF INTERMITTENT FASTING

Intermittent fasting is an eating design where you cycle between times of eating and fasting.

Autophagy or auto phagocytosis in extravagant science language deciphers from the Ancient Greek word autóphagos, which implies self-absorption or - eating up.

Autophagy is a characteristic procedure by which our cells dismantle and expel their useless parts. It's essentially the reusing of cell waste and taking out the rubbish.

Autophagy places you into a catabolic state, which stalls your own tissue, rather than an anabolic one, which is tied in with working up.
At the point when you trigger autophagy, you permit the organelles of your sound cells to chase out dead or infected cells and afterward eat them.

This includes shaping a twofold film around the phone that will be eaten called an autophagosome. The autophagosome then breaks down the wiped out cell or the harmful protein and makes vitality.

It doesn't utter a word about which foods to eat, yet rather when you ought to eat them.

There are a few distinctive intermittent fasting techniques, all of which split the day or week into eating periods and fasting periods.

The vast majority effectively "fast" consistently, while they rest. Intermittent fasting can be as straightforward as expanding that fast somewhat more.

You can do this by skipping breakfast, eating your first supper around early afternoon, and your last feast at 8 pm.

At that point, you're, in fact, fasting for 16 hours consistently, and limiting your eating to an 8-hour eating window. This is the most mainstream type of intermittent fasting, known as the 16/8 technique.

Regardless of what you may think, intermittent fasting is very simple to do. Numerous individuals report feeling good and having more vitality during a fast.

Appetite is normally not excessively huge of an issue, in spite of the fact that it very well may be an issue to start with, while your body is becoming accustomed to not eating for expanded timeframes.

No food is permitted during the fasting time frame, yet you can drink water, espresso, tea, and other non-caloric refreshments.

A few types of intermittent fasting permit modest quantities of low-calorie foods during the fasting time frame.

Taking enhancements is by and large permitted while fasting, as long as there are no calories in them.

Intermittent fasting (or "IF") is an eating design where you cycle between times of eating and fasting. It is a mainstream wellbeing and wellness pattern.

BENEFITS OF INTERMITTENT FASTING FOR WOMEN ABOVE 50

As women sail past 50, we will, in general, watch out for things that will improve our ageing experience, from serums and enhancements to diets, medications, and tenets. The items available are really interminable, however incidentally, perhaps the best thing you can accomplish for your ageing body doesn't include purchasing - or becoming tied up with - anything.

You may have known about intermittent fasting, which includes sensible, exchanging times of eating and not eating, otherwise known as fasting. Intermittent fasting is advantageous from multiple points of view, and this might be particularly valid for more established grown-ups.

Here are five benefits of intermittent fasting, alongside how to do it:

1. Intermittent fasting starts cell fix forms in your body.

Cell harm is good enough as we age, however, fasting has been appeared to prompt your body's cell fix forms, improve hormone work, and even improves the capacity of qualities identified with sickness insurance and life span.

2. Intermittent fasting advances weight loss- - particularly tummy fat.

Tummy fat means that instinctive fat, which lies somewhere inside the stomach cavity, encompassing your organs and adding to the ailment.

Losing paunch fat is intense, particularly as we age, however as per an ongoing writing audit, intermittent fasting can prompt a loss of four to seven per cent of your midsection periphery.

An ongoing report found that intermittent fasting can cause in general weight loss of three to eight percent more than three to 24 weeks.

3. Intermittent fasting diminishes aggravation and oxidative pressure.

Irritation and oxidative pressure are significant supporters of malady as we age, and they add to the noticeable indications of aging.

Intermittent fasting lessens markers of oxidative pressure and aggravation in overweight grown-ups, as per an examination by Louisiana State University Medical Center.

4. Intermittent fasting may help forestall Alzheimer's infection.

A huge body of research shows that intermittent fasting is useful for the brain, advancing the development of new nerve cells, shielding against brain harm coming about because of stroke, and expanding levels of a hormone called brain-determined neurotrophic factor or BDNF.

An ongoing report found that intermittent fasting likewise postponed the beginning of Alzheimer's or diminished its seriousness. Different investigations show that intermittent fasting may offer security against Parkinson's, Huntington's, and other neurodegenerative ailments.

5. Intermittent fasting may expand your life.

Intermittent fasting EXTENDS PEOPLE life expectancy.

These are some metabolic changes that IF causes that may help represent synergistic benefits:

- Insulin: During the fasting time frame, lower insulin levels will help improve fat burning.

- HGH: While insulin levels drop, HGH levels ascend to energize fat burning and muscle development.

- Noradrenaline: in light of an unfilled stomach, the sensory system will send this concoction to cells to tell them they have to discharge fat for fuel.

Intermittent fasting can accomplish more than assist individuals with getting thinner; it likewise may improve circulatory strain and help the body procedure fat.

Intermittent fasting could diminish the hazard for types of disease, yet more research is required.

There might be developmental reasons why denying ourselves of food for quite a while causes us to feel lively and centered.

"Hungry," from a developmental viewpoint, isn't dormant or depleted. It's the point at which our bodies and brains need to work at the most extreme limit.

"It bodes well that the brain should be working very well when an individual is in a fasted state since it's in that express that they need to make sense of how to discover food," Mattson revealed to Business Insider. "They likewise must have the option to use a great deal of vitality. People whose brains were not working admirably while fasting would not have the option to contend and flourish."

- Periodic fasting may cause it simpler for us to consume fat and enter ketosis.

Blood tests have indicated that individuals who fast from 12 to 24 hours one after another enter a state called ketosis — when their bodies begin to get more vitality from fat.

The more you enter this express, the better your body gets at utilizing fat as fuel. Hence, a few people attempt to trigger ketosis with "keto" counts calories that include expending a great deal of fat. In any case, as per Mattson, fasting is an essentially increasingly compelling method for boosting ketone levels.

- Intermittent fasting may reinforce neural associations and improve memory and mind-set.

- Human brain connectome

Numerous individuals who fast intermittently state that on occasion, they feel more clear and increasingly engaged while fasting.

There's genuine science to back up the possibility that being "ravenous" gives you a feeling of core interest. Entering ketosis triggers the arrival of an atom called BDNF, which reinforces neurons and brain associations connected to learning and memory.

That is one reason specialists have proposed that ketogenic slims down (both the fasting kind and the fat-substantial kind) could be helpful for individuals battling degenerative brain infections like Alzheimer's. That additionally could clarify the lucidity or concentrate a few people feel in the wake of fasting. It might give a state of mind helps too.

- Indicates that a few types of intermittent fasting may help with diabetes.

Both in mice and in individuals, there's proof that specific types of intermittent fasting can improve the body's reaction to sugar. In mice,

In individuals, a type of fasting that includes 25 days of unrestricted eating, followed by five days of eating a restricted fasting diet appears to cause huge upgrades for those with high glucose.
Intermittent fasting works at any rate just as different types of dieting for weight loss.

No type of confining food is essentially simple, and individuals who begin with intermittent fasting for the first time agreed that it's difficult. From one perspective, it's pleasant to eat whatever you need when your eating routine isn't restricted — but on the other hand, it's extremely difficult to realize you are still hours from food when hit with a hankering.

Intermittent fasting is in any event in the same class as different types of dieting for weight loss. That, in addition to the next medical advantages, may make it a favoured contender for some.

Some examination demonstrates that intermittent fasting may assist convert with bodying fat to dark-coloured fat, which assists ignite with offing overabundance weight.

Taking splits from food — accelerated the metabolism of mice. All the while, fat in their bodies was changed over to dark-coloured fat, a more advantageous kind of fat that helps consume with smouldering heat white fat, which is the thing that we consider as undesirable body fat that develops...

Certain types of fasting are related to antiaging wellbeing effects. However, it's uncertain whether intermittent fasting does this for people.

A few types of fasting have been related with essentially improved life expectancy and healthspan — the time a living being is sound — in a few investigations.

This has, for the most part, been shown with caloric limitation in creatures, which cuts the quantity of calories these creatures are given by somewhere in the range of 20% and 30%. There's restricted proof this may work for people as well.

Yet, that kind of fast doesn't sound essentially protected or wonderful.

It's hazy whether intermittent fasting would trigger similar benefits. However, it's conceivable.

It's engaging imagine that fasting may be an antiquated endurance system that triggers mending forms in the body.

Yet, that doesn't mean all types of fasting are the equivalent or that they have a similar wellbeing effect. Many will fluctuate from individual to individual, and you ought to consistently counsel your primary care physician before attempting any extreme dietary changes.

Know different types of fasts — like eating just during specific hours, limiting eating a couple of days seven days — are related to medical advantages. Yet, we don't have the foggiest idea about that all these medical advantages are the equivalent for all fasts.

In any case, all things being equal, a significant number of these intermittent-fasting regimens are generally considered ok for a sound individual. So on the off chance that they offer, they could merit a shot. What's more, they may accompany a large group of medical advantages.

TYPES OF INTERMITTENT FASTING

There are numerous reasons and methods for doing intermittent fasting, yet it's essential to separate a portion of the principle phrasing.

- Fasting – the demonstration of refusing food admission or anything that has calories for a specific timeframe. Typically, some non-caloric drinks and water are permitted.

- Intermittent Fasting – doing fasting intermittently and joining shorter fasts into your week by week plan.

- Extended Fasting – the demonstration of fasting for a drawn-out timeframe for extra medical advantages. It tends to be accomplished for quite a long time or even weeks.

- Time-Restricted Feeding – the demonstration of limiting your everyday food utilization inside a specific time window. This will improve circadian mood and general wellbeing.

By and large, individuals doing intermittent fasting are essentially time-limiting their food and not so much fasting. To classify something like a fast, it would need to keep going for more than 24 hours since that is the place the vast majority of the benefits begin to kick in.

It's straightforward – you simply quit eating – yet for ideal outcomes, you'd need to focus on these various types of intermittent fasting recorded beneath

#1. 24-Hour Fasting

This is the essential method for doing intermittent fasting – you fast for around 24 hours and afterwards have a meal. It doesn't need to imply that you really experience a day without eating. Just eat at night, fast all through the following day and have dinner once more.

You can even have your food at the 23-hour check and eat it inside 60 minutes. The thought is to force a greater caloric shortage for the afternoon and undereat. The majority of the benefits will be futile in the event that you despite everything gorge and put on weight.

To what extent and every now and again you can fastly rely upon your physical condition and vitality necessities.

• A fit individual who trains and exercises all the time would require somewhat increasingly visit eating and less fasting.

• An overweight individual who is inactive and attempts to lose some weight could fast as long as they can until they lose the overabundance weight.

Fasting and skipping dinners have gotten degenerate in the advanced food condition since you can eat anything anyplace. It's likewise the 'F-expression' of the wellness business. Be that as it may, fasting ought to be considered the most effortless and fastest method for getting in shape.

#2. 16/8 Intermittent Fasting

Individuals rehearsed the 16/8 style intermittent fasting a lot.

The 16:8 intermittent fasting was promoted by Martin Berkhan of Leangains. It's accomplished for enhancing fat loss while as yet having the option to prepare hard.

It's basic – you fast for 16 hours and eat your food inside 8. What number of suppers you have inside that time span is insignificant, yet anything else than 2-3 isn't important.

In my own view, this ought to be the base fasting length to focus on by everybody consistently. There is no physical motivation to eat any sooner than that, and the restraint has numerous benefits.

A great many people think that it is simpler to post-pone breakfast by a couple of hours and eat around early afternoon. You don't need to be psychotic, and that is exacting about breaking the fast The thought is just to lessen the measure of time we spend in a sustained state and too fastly most of the day.

#3. The Warrior Diet

The Warrior Diet is proposed by Ori Hofmekler. He gabs about the benefits of fasting on pressure adjustment through the wonder of hormesis.

Fasting not just improves your body's physical condition and capacity to endure upsetting conditions yet, in addition, sharpens your psychological mentality and mindset.

The Warrior Diet discusses old warriors like Spartans and Romans who might remain truly dynamic all throughout the whole day and eat for the most part at night. During light, they would walk around with 40 pounds of gear, manufacture fortifications, and bear the warming sun of the Mediterranean at the same time getting only a couple of chomps of food to a great extent. At night, they would have an enormous dinner contained stews, meat, pieces of bread, and different things.

On The Warrior Diet, you fast for around 20 hours, have a short high force exercise and eat your food inside 4 hours. By and large, it would incorporate either 2 littler dinners with a break in the middle of or one single huge dining experience.

#4 One Meal a Day OMAD

Perhaps the least difficult methods for eating is the One Meal a Day Diet or OMAD. You simply eat once every day, and it's finished.

On OMAD, you normally fast around 21-23 hours and eat your food inside a 1-2 hour timeframe. This is extraordinary for dieting since you can feel full and fulfilled while as yet remaining at a caloric shortfall.

OMAD is extraordinary for losing fat; however, not perfect for muscle development due to the constrained time for protein combination and anabolism. It's an extremely moderate procedure.

my involvement in intermittent fasting following 7 years of fasting

#5. 36-Hour Fasting

Previously, individuals would frequently go a few days without eating yet they endure and even flourished. These days, the normal individual can't skip breakfast, also head to sleep hungry.

Fasting for more than 24 hours is the place all the enchantment starts. The more you remain in a fasted state and experience vitality hardship, the more your body is compelled to trigger its life span pathways that help to activate fat stores, support immature microorganisms, and reuse old destroyed cell material through the procedure of autophagy.

For the most part, it takes, at any rate, a day to see huge indications of autophagy yet you can speed it up by eating low carb before beginning the fast, practising on an unfilled stomach, and expending some homegrown teas that animate this procedure.

Fasting for 36 hours isn't that troublesome really. You basically eat the earlier night, don't eat anything in the first part of the day, lunch nor evening, head to sleep in a fasted state, wake up the following day, fast a couple of hours more and begin eating once more.

Things that make the fasting simpler are shimmering water, mineral water, dark espresso, green tea, and some homegrown teas.

#6. 48-Hour Fasting

On the off chance that you previously made it to the 36-hour mark, at that point, why not simply fast for the whole 48 hours.

Fasting is just troublesome during the principal adjustment stage. After you cross the gorge, which for the most part, happens around your routine supper time, at that point, it gets very simple.

When your body goes into more profound ketosis and enacts autophagy, you will smother hunger, feel intellectually completely clear, and have more vitality and core interest.

The most troublesome piece of any all-inclusive fast is around the 24-hour mark. In the event that you can nod off and wake up the following day, at that point, you've set yourself ready for fasting for a considerable length of time and days without any issues. You simply need to get over this underlying hindrance.

Hitting the sack hungry sounds alarming; however, that is the thing that a large portion of the total populace is doing every day. It makes you ponder your own fortune and be progressively appreciative for your food.

#7. Extended Fasting for 3-7 Days

Fasting for 48 hours would give you a short lift in autophagy and some fat burning; however, to truly pick up the remedial benefits of fasting, you'd need to fast for 3+ days.

It's been demonstrated that 72-hours of fasting can reset the safe framework in mice]. This turns on pathways of undifferentiated hematopoietic organisms, which creates platelets and advances resistance.

Fasting for 3-5 days is additionally the ideal time period for autophagy also after which you start to see unavoidable losses. Fasting for 7 days and past isn't required by and large. Most individuals don't have to fast any more drawn out than that since you may begin losing fit muscle tissue.

Its fitting for individuals to focus on 3-4 of these all-encompassing fasts each year to advance cell recuperating and wipe out the body. In spite of eating a solid eating routine and not having any lousy nourishment, I despite everything do it in light of the stunning benefits.

On the off chance that you're overweight or you experience the ill effects of some ailment, at that point longer fasts can truly assist you with healing yourself. Fast for 3-5 days, have a little refeed, and rehash the procedure until important.

#8. Alternate Day Fasting

There are additionally moves toward like The 5:2 Diet and Alternate Day Fasting, which incorporate fasting, however, permit the utilization of around 500 calories on long periods of abstention. Those limited quantity of calories is just for expanding consistence.

Proceeding to eat at an extreme caloric limitation won't permit the entirety of the physiological benefits of fasting to kick in completely. You would increase a portion of the effects; however, a total restraint is significantly more compelling for both your physiology and brain science.

Conventions like the Fasting Mimicking Diet have their place, and they can be utilized now and again. Ordinarily, they're endorsed to individuals who aren't able to fast like the old or some therapeutic patients.

Physiologically everyone can fast. It's simply that some can't mentally deal with the pressure and to not eat. That is the place these fasting imitating diets and alternate-day fasting conventions can help.

#9. Fasting Mimicking Diet (FMD)

You eat around 800-1000 calories every day for 2-5 days of the month. At that point, you have a refeed day on day 6 and come back to a typical eating plan.

The fasting emulating diet has been appeared to lessen circulatory strain, lower insulin, and smother IGF-1, all of which have positive benefits on life span. In any case, these effects are likely a direct result of the extreme caloric limitation.

On the FMD, you'd eat low protein, moderate carb, moderate fat foods like mushroom soup, olives, kale wafers, and some nut bars. The thought is to, in any case, give you something to eat while keeping the calories as low as would be prudent. Be that as it may, once more, this is simply to fulfil the individuals mental want to eat.

Fasting with zero calories would be progressively successful, and it will really keep up more muscle tissue by remaining in more profound ketosis.

To forestall undesirable loss of lean mass, you can alter the macronutrient proportions of the FMD and make them more ketogenic by bringing down the carbs and expanding the fat marginally.

#10. Protein Sparing Modified Fasting

The protein-sparing modified fast (PSMF) is a low carb, low fat, high protein kind of diet that assists with getting more fit truly fast while advancing muscle upkeep.

Keeping slender bulk is a major matter of worry for individuals who are into wellness, particularly on the off chance that they're attempting to do intermittent fasting.

Fasting is a catabolic stressor that will, in the long run, lead to muscle loss; however, the rate is a lot of lower than individuals might suspect. To keep that from occurring, you need to remain in ketosis and lower the body's interest for glucose. At the point when ketones are available, the prerequisite for separating muscle into vitality diminishes fundamentally.
The PSMF is certainly going to keep up more muscle than the fasting mirroring diet yet there's the threat of being kicked out of ketosis on the off chance that you eat an excess of protein in this manner pre-arranging yourself to muscle catabolism.

To stay away from muscle loss on the protein-sparing modified fast, you need to keep protein moderate around 0.8-1.0 g/lb of body weight and increment your fat a tad. Altogether, you'd even now remain under 1000 calories for each day.

#11. Fat Fasting

The physiology of fasting and the ketogenic diet are fundamentally the same as, and the two of them initiate the metabolic condition of ketosis.

At the point when you're in ketosis, you're utilizing fat and ketones as an essential fuel source rather than glucose. This empowers you to gain admittance to vitality day in and day out on the grounds that you'll be burning your own body fat.

Expending just fat during a fast ala fat fasting won't show you out of ketosis. It likely raises your ketones marginally. Be that as it may, it will stifle autophagy a tad.

A few types of autophagy like chaperone-mediated autophagy can rescue ketones and keep up their effects; however, it's not as powerful as macroautophagy, which requires the forbearance from all calories.

A fat fast can be utilized for advancing adherence and ensuring you don't stop partially through.

During fat fasting, you can have a touch of Bulletproof espresso, 1-2 tsp of MCT oil, or some margarine however anything with carbs or protein in it like bone broth, coconut milk, overwhelming cream, coconut water, or the like will break the fast.

#12 Bone Broth Fasting

Bone broth fasting is as yet a reasonable alternative for broadened fasting on the off chance that it causes you unreasonably fast for more.

Bone broth has some amino acids in it that actually can repress autophagy yet on the off chance that you just beverage a solitary cup, at that point you'll most likely stifle autophagy for only a couple of hours and get again into it fastly.

On the off chance that you're doing fasting for autophagy, at that point, you need to utilize bone broth and different calories if all else fails not to destroy them fast.

For fat loss, you would prefer not to be expending a lot of calories either on the grounds that it won't be justified, despite all the trouble. A solitary cup of broth at the most troublesome piece of the fast can assist you with overcoming it yet anything else than that makes you basically expend more calories in this way hindering the weight loss.

The electrolytes and minerals in bone broth are additionally incredible for forestalling brain mist, laziness, and dodging muscle cramps.

#13. Dry Fasting

Not drinking fluids is additionally said to have autophagic benefits. One day of dry fasting is thought to rise to 3 days of water fasting.

The thought is that in the event that you deny yourself from water, your body will begin to deliver its own by changing over the triglycerides from the fat tissue into metabolic water. Hydrogen gets discharged as a result of beta-oxidation.

Dry fasting has been polished in certain strict and mending rehearses. As a rule, you would prefer not to get got dried out for a really long time. In any case, every day time-restricted dry fasting of 12-16 hours can be something else to do on the off chance that you need further autophagy.

At your own hazard, obviously.

#14. Juice Fasting

There are additionally some juice fasting conventions where you just beverage juices and smoothies. Actually, it could work similarly of the fasting impersonating diet yet by and by it's not justified, despite any potential benefits.

Squeezing vegetables and natural product causes you to expend a serious critical measure of starches and fructose, which will all meddle with both ketosis and autophagy very hard.

You can lose a lot of weight with juice fasting, yet a large portion of it will be muscle and other fit tissue. That is the reason you need and should be in ketosis to make the fast protected.

Regardless of whether you're utilizing things like just kale or spinach to make a smoothie, you'd most likely log jam the mending of fasting as a result of the high measures of fibre.

In the event that you need to smother hunger or have something to drink that doesn't pose a flavour like water, at that point have some simmering water with 2 tsp of apple juice vinegar. It won't stop the fast and really has extraordinary medical advantages.

#15. Time-Restricted Feeding

Time-Restricted Feeding developed as an idea after the advancement of circadian rhythms and chronobiology. Basically, you essentially a time limit your day by day food utilization.

Time-restricted sustaining has likewise been appeared to forestall metabolic disarranges in mice who are encouraged a high-fat eating regimen without decreasing calories. The mice who have sustained their food inside 8 hours didn't get stout or create sickness contrasted with the individuals who ate a similar measure of calories with no time limitations. This shows the demonstration of essentially time-confining your food admission has significant benefits on general wellbeing and body structure. The distinction might be little, yet it's still there.

The contrast between intermittent fasting and time-restricted sustaining is that one is done intermittently, for example, the 36 hour fast while the other ought to be a piece of your day by day eating plan.

DIFFERENCES BETWEEN THE TYPES OF INTERMITTENT FASTING

The principle comparability is the act of restraint from food and drink. The distinction anyway lies in the point and rationale behind fasting-one being for strict and profound reasons, and the other being to shed weight.

Underlying foundations of fasting: A ton of what we call 'intermittent fasting' these days originates from observational research dependent on Ramadan practices and results.

Fasting is an old practice followed in a wide range of configurations by populaces all-inclusive dependent on religion or culture, however more as of late in the medicinal world too for wellbeing reasons.

"As of now, there is really an insufficient proof for us to recognize what the perfect number of fasting hours ought to be to advance results.

Types of intermittent fasting There are four fundamental types of intermittent fasting that fluctuate in term and calorie admission. These incorporate alternate-day fasting, entire day fasting, modified fasting systems, and time-restricted sustaining.

"Stars of intermittent fasting are that numerous individuals see it as an increasingly adaptable methodology, that doesn't require the exact following of calories and less arranging is required.

Studies have likewise demonstrated that intermittent fasting can be as successful for weight loss as a proceeded with the calorie-restricted eating regimen.

WHY THE INTERMITTENT FASTING IS FOR WOMEN OVER 50

Women more than 50 face issues, for example, lower bulk, trouble in dozing, throbbing joints, and a more slow metabolism.

Intermittent fasting for women more than 50 is really an incredible healing strategy as it assists ward with offing or limits almost all the age-related issues you face more than 50. It additionally assists withholding your weight within proper limits.

A major piece of the accomplishment of intermittent fasting lays in getting aware of food utilization. You will think that its simple to maintain a strategic distance from unfortunate foods, including handled carbs, void calories, and fats. Joining intermittent fasting with different weight control plans likewise assists with upgrading the impact of the eating routine.

The general benefits that persuade women towards taking up intermittent fasting include:

- Enhanced fit muscle development

- Increase in vitality

- Continuous weight loss

- An increased cell stress response

- Reduced aggravation and oxidative pressure

- Improvement in insulin affectability in women who are overweight

- Enhanced intellectual capacity because of expanded nerve development factor creation

In any case, besides all the benefits, there are sure considerations to think about.

The first is the fasting stage that causes the creation of leptin and ghrelin – the appetite hormones. Be that as it may, as women give intermittent fasting some time, they report feeling less ravenous over the long haul.

The second factor in intermittent fasting for women is the fasting hinders the regenerative limit, so it isn't prescribed for pregnant women to fast. In the event that a lady who fasts neglects to devour enough calories, she may have some richness issues. Be that as it may, if is done accurately, there's no compelling reason to stress. In the wake of losing some overweight women may even improve their richness.

DIFFERENCES OF INTERMITTENT FASTING BETWEEN YOUNG AND OLD FOR BODY ILLNESS AND HEALING

Ailment, mending, sport

The upsides of intermittent fasting for women are settled and science-sponsored. However, for what reason is it explicitly gainful for women more than 50?

1.   Weight Loss

Weight loss is among the top benefits of intermittent fasting for women more than 50, contrasted with youngsters. There are declarations wherever about how intermittent fasting has helped individuals lose substantial measures of weight. There are additionally scholastic investigations that help this thought.

2.   Lowering Cancer Risk

In the event that has demonstrated to be a significant prognostic apparatus against malignancy. The underlying proof has discovered that the demonstration of fasting restrains certain pathways that may somehow or another lead to the improvement and movement of malignant growth.

3.   Reducing Diabetes Risk

The danger of diabetes, which especially elevates during middle age, can be effectively controlled through intermittent fasting. It does as such by bringing down insulin level and controlling insulin opposition in the body.

4.   Anti-ageing

On the off chance that has been accounted for to hinder the improvement of infections that lead to death. Intermittent fasting for women more than 50 can assist them with carrying on with a more extended, more beneficial life when contrasted with the individuals who follow a normal eating regimen plan.

5.   Heart Health

It is typical for your cardiovascular wellbeing to begin declining around age 40. On the off chance that can help hinder this weakening and forestall certain cardiovascular infections like hypertension by bringing down LDL cholesterol and triglycerides.

6.   Reduced Inflammation

Constant irritation harms your body, making it harder to get thinner.

Following intermittent fasting, nonetheless, turns around irritation and may improve your general prosperity.

7.   Muscle Preservation

One of the benefits of following IF is that it encourages you to lose more weight while holding bulk. A higher bulk, thus, encourages you to consume more calories, in any event, when you are not engaged with physical exercises.

8.   Decreased Cravings

Another advantage of intermittent fasting for women more than 40 is diminished yearnings. Changing to this eating routine modifies your dietary patterns and normally assist you with eating lesser than expected. This reductions the quantity of calories devoured every day and therefore, diminishes body weight.

9.   Improvement in Mental Health

In the event that in females have been getting a kick out of the chance to neurogenesis: the procedure where new brain cells are delivered. Neurogenesis, at last, expands your brain execution, centre, state of mind, and memory.

Different benefits of intermittent fasting for women more than 50 may include:

- Sustainable weight loss

- An increment in slender bulk

- More vitality

- An increment in cell stress reaction

- A decrease in oxidative pressure and aggravation

- Improvement around insulin affectability in overweight women

- Increased generation of neurotrophic development factor (which could support psychological capacity)

Presently, here's the dubious part. Albeit intermittent fasting may have its benefits, women are normally touchy to indications of starvation, so intermittent fasting for women is an entire diverse monster.

At the point when the female body detects it's going towards starvation, it will build the creation of the yearning hormones, ghrelin and leptin, which signal the body that you're ravenous and need to eat. Also, if there's insufficient food for you to endure, your body will close down the framework that would permit you to make another human. This is the body's common method for ensuring a potential pregnancy, regardless of whether you're not really pregnant or attempting to imagine.

While some nutrition specialists fight that IF works since it helps individuals normally limit food admission, others oppose this idea. They accept that intermittent fasting results are superior to anything run of the mill feast plans with a similar measure of calories and different supplements. Studies have even proposed that keeping away from food for a few hours daily accomplishes something other than limit the measure of calories you expend.

These are some metabolic changes that IF causes that may help represent synergistic benefits:

• Insulin: During the fasting time frame, lower insulin levels will help improve fat burning.

• HGH: While insulin levels drop, HGH levels ascend to energize fat burning and muscle development.

• Noradrenaline: in light of an unfilled paunch, the sensory system will send this compound to cells to tell them they have to discharge fat for fuel.

Is Intermittent Fasting Healthy?

Is intermittent fasting safe? Recall that you're just expected to fast for twelve to sixteen hours and not for a considerable length of time at once. You've, despite everything got a lot of time to appreciate a fantastic and sound eating routine. Obviously, some more seasoned women may need to eat often due to metabolic scatters or the directions on solutions. All things considered, you ought to examine your dietary patterns with your restorative supplier before rolling out any improvements.

While it's not in fact fasting, a few specialists have announced intermittent fasting benefits by permitting such simple to-process food as an entirely natural product during the fasting window. Alterations like these can, in any case, give your stomach related and metabolic framework a required rest. For instance, "Fit forever" was a famous weight loss book that proposed eating just organic product after dinner and before lunch.

Indeed, the writers of this book said that they had patients who just changed their dietary patterns with this twelve-to sixteen-hour "organic product" fast every day. They didn't adhere to the eating routine's different guidelines or check calories, they despite everything shed pounds and got more beneficial. This technique may have just worked in light of the fact that the weight watchers supplanted low-quality nourishment with entire foods. Regardless, individuals discovered this dietary change compelling and simple to make. Conventionalists won't call this fasting; be that as it may, realize that you may have choices on the off chance that you completely can't go without food for a few hours one after another.

While the vast majority intend to take up intermittent fasting for weight loss, it's not only for weight watchers. It offers a huge number of medical advantages that gives the majority of our motivations to give it a go!

Not at all like a consistent low-calorie diet or an outrageous eating regimen that expects you to remove certain food bunches like sugars inside and out, intermittent fasting sprinkles typical eating with a feast avoided from time to time. It could likewise mean a day or two of fasting in the middle of normal days.

Also, fasting doesn't need to be a tough assignment. Truth be told, when you rest each night, you are — as a result, permitting your body to fast for the 8 hours that you rest and until you eat. The ongoing examination has discovered that intermittent fasting offers a scope of medical advantages. So what are these benefits?

1. Fat Burning and Weight Loss

Expanded fat burning is the most evident advantage of intermittent fasting. At the point when you go on a fast, your body's glucose and insulin levels drop altogether. Without glucose, the body goes to fat burning. One little investigation of non-fat people found that fat oxidation rates expanded after alternate-day fasting.1

Human development hormone levels likewise rise fundamentally in the wake of fasting.

This hormone is said to help with fat burning just as muscle gain. Intermittent fasting can build slender body mass and cut down fat mass in sound seniors of the two sexual orientations.

Intermittent fasting can support

- Basal metabolic rate by 3.6%

- Resting vitality use by 14%

- Fat loss by 4%–7%

- Weight loss by 3%–8%

Unavoidably, this prompts weight loss. In the first place, since you're eating less dinners, it lessens your everyday calorie utilization. Second, it expands your basal metabolism – the rate at which you consume calories when very still. Fasting totally (starvation) for 48 hours made basal metabolism of the subjects ascend by about 3.6% on a normal.

The metabolic rate, as estimated by resting vitality consumption, rose by around 14% on the principal day of a multi-day (84-hour) fast. This change in metabolic rate could be on the grounds that, as referenced prior, fasting improves the working of development hormones. It additionally builds the measure of the hormone norepinephrine, which supports fat burning, and these variables assume a job in the breakdown of body fat.

Subsequently, intermittent fasting may permit you to profit by this raised metabolic rate to consume off calories – without fasting for significant stretches of time. Truth be told, one examination led on type 2 diabetics found that intermittent fasting can assist individuals with losing up to 3–8% of body weight and 4–7% of fat from their midriff through the span of 3–24 weeks!

2. Improves Diabetes Symptoms

Diabetics could profit by intermittent fasting if they do it under restorative supervision. Intermittent fasting has been found to:

•	Hike insulin affectability: Diabetics ordinarily experience the ill effects of low insulin affectability, which prompts high insulin just as glucose levels in the blood. Overabundance insulin is additionally destructive over the long haul. In an examination, male members who fasted intermittently noticed a decrease in their glucose levels by 3–6% and in their fasting insulin levels by 20–31%.

•	Regenerate beta cells in the pancreas: Type 1 diabetics have not very many insulin-creating beta cells in their pancreas, which is the thing that causes diabetes. Fasting intermittently can even assistance recover the insulin-creating beta cells in the pancreas.

•	Prevent diabetes inconveniences: This type of fasting forestalled kidney harm, a typical diabetes confusion.

Keep in mind, and the key is too fast "intermittently." If you continually go on a fast, you may really wind up with progressively stomach fat because of impeded morning glucose resistance and postponed insulin reaction.

3. Lessens Inflammation

Irritation is the body's regular (insusceptible) reaction to damage and remote trespassers, (for example, infections and microorganisms). Notwithstanding, ceaseless aggravation has been associated with various sicknesses that plague individuals today –, for example, joint pain, diabetes, coronary illness, Alzheimer's, and malignant growth.

Besides bringing down irritation, by keeping up brain structure and capacity, intermittent fasting is accepted to ease interminable torment.

At the point when you fast, your body discharges ghrelin, the appetite hormone, which is known to bring down aggravation and help in the treatment of any ailments related with it. Furthermore, intermittent fasting diminishes the quantity of provocative proteins called cytokines. Also, considering how fasting for only one feast can have any kind of effect, intermittent fasting is frequently suggested for individuals with provocative disarranges.

4. Forestalls Heart Diseases

Alternate-day fasting has been found to help decrease levels of triglycerides while improving degrees of good high-thickness lipoprotein (HDL) cholesterol. Both these elements are fundamental in securing the heart. Likewise, intermittent fasting brings down circulatory strain and resting pulse similarly as serious exercise does. While a steady circulatory strain advances cardiovascular wellbeing, a lower pulse very still shows better heart work and cardiovascular wellness.

5. Brings down Risk Of Metabolic Diseases

Time-restricted sustaining can help forestall metabolic infections like liver ailment and heftiness even on a high-fat eating routine. This could be on the grounds that fasting improves cell flagging (correspondence among cells) and builds metabolism. It does not shock anyone then that specialists have been prescribing intermittent fasting to people with metabolic maladies.

6. Improves Digestion

Fasting boosts the generation of the hormone ghrelin, the appetite hormone. This hormone assumes a significant job in processing and gut wellbeing. It readies the body for supplement assimilation by emitting gastric corrosive and invigorating the developments of liquids in the gastrointestinal framework. This could be the reason fasting has been appeared to improve indications like stomach agony, loose bowels, and sickness brought about by colitis, ischemia, and peevish entrail disorder.

7. May Improve Sleep

As per a source, you are not eating anything for 16 hours before awakening could improve rest quality.

In the event that you will in general thrash around evening time and get up each morning very drowsy and restless, you may profit by intermittent fasting. It improves the nature of rest and diminishes the occasions one awakens in the night.

Be that as it may, individuals who practise intermittent fasting may encounter restlessness and daytime sluggishness as a side impact. Since there are blended outcomes on the effects of intermittent fasting on rest, it's ideal to counsel a specialist first, particularly on the off chance that you are under treatment for a sleeping disorder.

8. Advances Skin Health

Intermittent fasting may expand the pace of twisted mending as well as lessen unfavourably susceptible responses (on the skin) and skin break out.

There is some proof that joins intermittent fasting to faster twisted mending.

Be that as it may, this isn't the main advantage that this type of fasting carries with it. It can help in lightening contact dermatitis and interminable urticarial – unfavourably susceptible responses on the skin. It is accepted that fasting intermittently can likewise lessen skin inflammation breakouts, yet there isn't sufficient research to back this up.

9. Boosts Mood and Motivation

In the event that you've been feeling low generally, you could attempt intermittent fasting. Since it improves rest, this type of fasting is additionally connected to an expansion in inspiration and better daytime execution as a rule errands. Devouring less calories and fasting intermittently has likewise appeared to bring down sorrow and improve disposition in ageing men. This could be because of the way that intermittent fasting boosts ghrelin, which is connected to the hippocampus, the piece of the brain that is liable for feeling.

10. Advances Brain Health

Learning may be the best when one fasts during the day since this is when ghrelin levels are high. Ghrelin recovers brain cells.

Intermittent fasting can likewise advance brain wellbeing. For example, this type of fasting could help ensure you against the effects of hereditary and natural factors that assume a job in the ageing of the brain and any related fragility, for example, muscle loss. This type of fasting is additionally connected with the development of the hippocampus, the piece of the brain that is liable for feeling and memory.

Besides this, Regular intermittent fasting improved memory and learning.
11. May Prevent Alzheimer's, Parkinson's, And Huntington's Disease

Fasting has been believed to support the creation of a protein called BDNF, which thusly advances the generation of neurons. This may counter nerve-deteriorating maladies like Alzheimer's.

Neurodegenerative illnesses don't have a fix, which is the reason forestalling them is basic. Researchers interface the overaction of nerves to deteriorating sicknesses like Alzheimer's Parkinson's, and Huntington's ailment.

Primer examinations express that intermittent fasting may:

• Slow down the beginning of Parkinson's illness by expanding the creation of ghrelin, the craving hormone. This hormone expands the convergence of dopamine in a piece of the brain where the decrease of dopamine cells causes Parkinson's malady.

• Delay the beginning of Alzheimer's malady or decrease its seriousness.

• Daily transient fasts improved the side effects of Alzheimer's in 9 out of 10 patients.

•   Delay the beginning of Huntington's infection and increment the life expectancy of patients.

12. Lightens Asthma Symptoms

You could lighten asthma indications by simply avoiding one supper of 400–500 calories each alternate day.

As expressed before, intermittent fasting lessens aggravation and oxidative worry in the body. Furthermore, this, thusly, can improve the side effects of asthma, particularly in individuals who are overweight. This applies to those with milder types of asthma. Avoiding only one supper of around 400–500 calories each other day could diminish challenges in relaxing.

13. Battles Infections

Fasting boosts the generation of neutrophils, a kind of white platelets, and immunoglobulin An, an antibody that assumes a basic job in a safe capacity. This enables your body to fend off contaminations by microorganisms like Salmonella.

Intermittent fasting has likewise demonstrated guarantee in forestalling harm to the brain over the span of contamination.

14. May Improve Symptoms of Autoimmune Diseases

Fasting intermittently is accepted to bring down the immune system reaction and advance the recovery of resistant cells.

This type of fasting may turn around the indications of different sclerosis, lupus, and vacuities.

Intermittent fasting as a method of managing immune system infections.

15. Forestalls Cancer

Fasting each alternate day or fasting for longer interims during the night may forestall disease.

We definitely realize that intermittent fasting brings down blood glucose levels. It additionally brings down degrees of the hormone IGF-1 (insulin-like development factor) in the body. These together add to a lower danger of malignancy.

It additionally lowers the occurrence of malignancy in the wake of fasting each alternate day.

To add to this, diminishing one's caloric admission and fasting for longer interims during the night has been found to decrease the danger of bosom malignant growth.

16. Expands Lifespan

Intermittent fasting may stretch out your life expectancy by up to 30%.

Considering the scope of medical advantages that have just been recorded, it's nothing unexpected that intermittent fasting is known to expand one's life expectancy. For one, it defers ageing by shielding the body from sickness. It likewise takes a shot at the natural pathways that drag out the wellbeing range of the sensory system. Besides this, intermittent fasting boosts the body's pressure obstruction, which expands the life span.

Those that fasted normally lived 83% longer than rodents that didn't.

Intermittent fasting can build an individual's life expectancy by up to 30%.

Pick Among The 5 Types Of Intermittent Fasting

- 16:8 – Fast for 16 hours, eat everything you can in 8 hours.

- 5:2 – Fast for 2 days per week, eat for 5 days.

- Alternate-day – Fast every alternate day.

- Warrior diet – Fast during the day, eat around evening time.

- Eat stop eat – Fast for 24 hours a few times per week.

Be that as it may, Take Caution! Intermittent Fasting Is NOT For Everyone

Fasting of any sort is best attempted under the direction of a certified dietician or nutritionist who can assist you with your dinner arranging. In any event, something as apparently innocuous as intermittent fasting that includes skirting only one feast from time to time could be risky for certain individuals. Here are a few cases where fasting without supervision is definitely not a smart thought:

- If you are pregnant

- If you are diabetic or have insulin obstruction or other glucose guideline issues

- If you have any sort of dietary issue

- If you don't rest soundly

- If you have some other medical issue that could jeopardize your life or intensify your condition in the event that you skipped dinners or didn't eat at customary interims

- If you are not a grown-up – youngsters with developing bodies have diverse nutritional needs and more dynamic ways of life than most grown-ups. Intermittent fasting is likely not a smart thought. In the event that it is something required for strict reasons, it is best finished with most extreme consideration and with cautious arranging and under the direction and with the assent of their folks.

HOW TO START INTERMITTENT FASTING FOR WOMEN OVER 50

Intermittent fasting for women is a successful weight loss approach, particularly women more than 50. As women age, getting more fit turns out to be increasingly testing. Intermittent fasting gives a simple method for women to shed pounds and accomplish extraordinary wellbeing. This book will detail the particular benefits of intermittent fasting for women more than 50.

It very well may be somewhat extraordinary because of an adjustment in your hormones and proteins that you don't understand immediately. On the off chance that you have been attempting to get more fit and you are 50 or more established, you most likely definitely realize that it isn't as simple as it once been.

Best food and beverages for intermittent fasting

Drink liquids: Drink a lot of water during your fast, and as you end your fast, centre around refreshments like milk, organic product squeezes or mixed beverages like smoothies. These will, in general, be a delicate method for getting your body some nutrition — they contain copper, manganese, potassium and fibre — without over-burdening the stomach related procedure. That said; attempt to maintain a strategic distance from sugar-substantial beverages.

Eat dried foods: Dates are a conventional fast breaking food in the Islamic confidence, and they give starches and micronutrients, as well. Other dried natural products that give sugar and fibre, like dried apricots or raisins, are acceptable fast breaking foods also.

Taste on soup: Another customary food, brothy soups help to keep you hydrated. Search for soups that have protein, similar to beans or lentils and carbs like pasta or rice.

Pick solid foods: If you think fasting implies that when you're eating once more, it's a free-for-all, reconsider — keeping your post-fast suppers solid, as well. They'll sound commonplace: natural product, vegetables, entire grains, lentils, solid fats and lean protein.

The food list for protein include:

- Poultry and fish

- Eggs

- Seafood

- Dairy items, for example, milk, yoghurt, and cheddar

- Seeds and nuts

- Beans and vegetables

- Soy

- Whole grains

The intermittent fasting food list for hydration include:

- Water

- Sparkling water

- Black espresso or tea

- Watermelon

- Strawberries

- Cantaloupe

- Peaches

- Oranges

- Skim milk

- Lettuce

- Cucumber

- Celery

- Tomatoes

- Plain yoghurt

Foods to eat from the Intermittent Fasting Food List

- Processed foods

- Refined grains

- Trans-fat

- Sugar-improved drinks

- Candy bars

- Processed meat

- Alcoholic drinks

Drinks can be a lifeline with regards to warding off food cravings and longings during your fasting windows. There are even sure beverages that can help improve the benefits of your intermittent fasting plan. Sweet!

Here are 5 beverages to appreciate during your fasting windows:

1. Water

You can (and should!) unquestionably drink water during your fasting windows. Water is constantly an extraordinary decision throughout the day, consistently. It tends to be still or shimmering, whatever you appreciate. On the off chance that you incline toward lemon water, you can likewise include a crush of lemon (or lime) to your water. For other enjoyment enhance varieties, take a stab at imbuing a pitcher of water with cucumber or orange cuts.

In any case, ensure you avoid any misleadingly improved water enhancers (like Crystal Light). The fake sugar can meddle with your fast.

2. Espresso

Dark espresso is a sans calorie refreshment that doesn't influence insulin levels. You can drink customary espresso (juiced) or decaf espresso during fasting windows, simply don't include any sugar or milk. Flavours like cinnamon are absolutely fine!

Numerous espresso consumers appreciate a cup of joe, or even coffee, during fasting windows with no antagonistic effects. Yet, a few people experience a dashing heart or agitated stomach on the off chance that they drink espresso during fasting windows, so screen your own understanding.

Reward: dark espresso may really improve a portion of the benefits of intermittent fasting, and it's very famous with individuals who likewise follow a keto diet. This showed taking in caffeine can bolster ketone generation. Espresso has additionally been appeared to help sound glucose levels over the long haul.

3. Bone Broth

Bone broth (or vegetable broth) is prescribed for whenever you choose to fast for 24 hours or more.

Be careful with canned broths or bouillon 3D shapes! These have huge amounts of fake flavours and additives that will balance the effects of your fast. A decent handcrafted broth, or one made by a confided in the source, is the best approach.

4. Tea

Help increment your satiety normally with tea! It very well might be a distinct advantage that, makes your fasting arrangement simpler as well as progressively effective. Peruse our introduction on the best way to utilize tea to upgrade your intermittent fasting plan.

A wide range of tea is extraordinary to drink during a fast, including green, dark, oolong and natural teas. Tea boosts the adequacy of intermittent fasting by supporting gut wellbeing, probiotic balance, and cell wellbeing.

Green tea, specifically, has been demonstrated to help increment satiety and bolster solid weight the board.

5. Apple Cider Vinegar

Drinking apple juice vinegar has various medical advantages, and you can keep drinking it while intermittent fasting, in any event, during fasting windows. Furthermore, since ACV assists with supporting solid glucose and assimilation, it might even improve the effects of your intermittent fasting plan.

On the off chance that you aren't an enthusiast of the apple juice vinegar drink, attempt it as serving of mixed greens dressing during eating windows. It's beneficial for you whenever of the day!

Risks and when ought to evade intermittent fasting

Intermittent fasting is by all accounts, the new pattern whirling among society. Intermittent fasting is a foreordained period that an individual intentionally doesn't eat food. There is a wide range of sorts of fasting strategies, much the same as there are numerous sorts of diets. From the 12-hour fast to the alternate day fasting, there are numerous sorts of fasts that are getting progressively well known. The idea behind intermittent fasting is that after the body is exhausted of sugars, it begins to consume fat around 12-24 hours after starvation so along these lines keeping the body from food for 12-24 hours will conceivably prompt weight loss which can improve wellbeing. Notwithstanding, the greater part of the examinations done on this theme have been performed on creatures over a brief period and have estimated glucose levels as opposed to long haul wellbeing results. Many contend that intermittent fasting isn't really perilous, however numerous likewise concur that intermittent fasting isn't alright for everybody. So truly, it is conceivable to lose calories, fat and weight from this well-known eating regimen anyway it is additionally conceivable to similarly as fast recover the weight, grow low vitality stores which can bring about a discouraged state of mind, issues resting and even organ harm if the fasting is extraordinary. Coming up next are reasons why people ought to keep away from intermittent fasting:

People who are underweight, battling with weight increase, under 18 years old, pregnant, or who are breastfeeding ought not to endeavour an intermittent fasting diet, as they need adequate calories consistently for legitimate advancement.

You ought to abstain from fasting inside and out on the off chance that you are in danger of a dietary problem.

Intermittent fasting has a high relationship with bulimia nervosa, and subsequently, people who are vulnerable to a dietary issue ought not to experience any eating routine related to fasting. Hazard factors for a dietary issue incorporate having a relative with a dietary issue, hairsplitting, impulsivity and state of mind shakiness.

You will in all likelihood feel hungry, indulge, become dried out, feel tired and be bad-tempered

Intermittent fasting isn't for weak-willed, implying that regardless of whether you are not underweight, you are more than 18 years old, you are not inclined to a dietary problem, and you are not pregnant or breastfeeding you will doubtlessly have some undesirable side effects.

- You will undoubtedly see your stomach is protesting during fasting periods, fundamentally in the event that you are utilized to steady touching for the duration of the day. To keep away from these appetite torments during fasting periods, abstain from taking a gander at, smelling, or in any event, pondering food, which can trigger the arrival of gastric corrosive into your stomach and cause you to feel hungry.

- Non-fasting days are not days when you can spend lavishly on anything you desire as this can prompt weight gain. Fasting may likewise prompt an expansion in the pressure hormone, cortisol, which may prompt considerably more food desires. Remember that indulging and voraciously consuming food is two basic side effects of intermittent fasting.

- Intermittent fasting is now and again connected with lack of hydration since when you don't eat, some of the time you neglect to drink, so it is basic to effectively remain hydrated for the duration of the day by drinking, overall, three litres of water.

- You will in all probability feel tired in light of the fact that your body is running on less vitality than expected, and since fasting can help feelings of anxiety, it can likewise upset your rest designs. In this manner, it is significant to receive a sound, ordinary rest example and stick to it so you can feel laid on a regular premise.

- The same natural chemistry that directs the state of mind additionally manages craving with supplement utilization influencing the movement of synapses like dopamine and serotonin, which assume a job in nervousness and gloom.

  That implies deregulating your hunger may do likewise to your disposition, and along these lines, you will in all likelihood feel fractious on events when you are fasting.

- The last recommendation for people who are keen on an intermittent fasting diet it constrains your liquor consumption just during eating periods. Try not to drink liquor during or following fasting and regardless of whether you drink during your eating periods, remember that drinking liquor implies that you are uprooting your chance for satisfactory nutrition.

At the point when you ought to keep away from intermittent fasting;

For certain individuals, intermittent fasting (IF) is a finished distinct advantage. It's the way to everything from manageable weight loss to expanded mental lucidity to a genuine lift in vitality.

Be that as it may, in light of the fact that intermittent fasting is the go-to way of life for certain individuals doesn't imply that it's for everybody. While intermittent fasting is a solid decision for a few, for other people, it can really be hazardous.

In any case, who precisely ought to keep away from intermittent fasting? What is a portion of the perils? Furthermore, what are a few choices for individuals who aren't an ideal choice for intermittent fasting—yet need to receive comparable rewards?

Insulin-Dependent Diabetics

One populace that could put themselves at genuine hazard by following an intermittent fasting plan? Individuals who battle with Type1 or insulin-subordinate diabetes.

"Intermittent fasting cycles between times of fasting and unrestricted eating. In individuals living with diabetes and who take antidiabetic prescriptions, particularly insulin, this could be extremely hazardous,"

"Anti-diabetic prescriptions, explicitly insulin, will keep on affecting glucose on the fasting days. This could drop sugar levels to a perilous point," she includes.

Diabetics need to keep up stable glucose levels to remain solid (through both eating routine and exercise). This can be about inconceivable with intermittent fasting.

Notwithstanding a sound eating regimen, practice is likewise significant.

Perseverance Athletes

Preparing for a long-distance race or an up and coming Ironman? Assuming this is the case, intermittent fasting likely isn't for you.

"Supplement timing is critical for sports execution and would be a test while following an intermittent fasting diet,"

"Continuance sports require expanded calorie needs as a result of the abundance of calories consumed. Furthermore, the effect [that] continuance practice has on supplement needs previously, during, and after an occasion or long instructional meeting requires reliable calorie admission and satisfactory macronutrient admission to fix muscle, recharge glycogen stores, and keep up electrolyte balance."

Intermittent fasting doesn't give you the relentless portion of calories and supplements you have to prepare, perform, and recuperate. In this way, in the event that you have a perseverance occasion coming up, you should plan to maintain a strategic distance from intermittent fasting.

Individuals with a History of Disordered Eating

In case you're recuperating from confused eating practices, intermittent fasting is a no-go. "A few people who will need to maintain a strategic distance from intermittent fasting incorporate those with a propensity to confused eating or a history of a dietary problem,"

Intermittent fasting requires times of limitation followed by times of eating bigger dinners. This can be incredibly activating for individuals who battle with confining, gorging, or other cluttered eating designs. In such cases, it's better for women above 50 to maintain a strategic distance from intermittent fasting out and out and adhere to a progressively steady nutrition plan.

Pregnant Women

At the point when you're conveying a kid, you have to follow a pregnancy diet that is loaded up with supplements (and calories!) to keep you and your child sound. Sadly, you won't get that with intermittent fasting.

"Individuals with interminable conditions, for example, diabetes or malignant growth, would not have any desire to rehearse intermittent fasting due to the potential for low glucose, lacking calorie consumption, and the chance of not meeting satisfactory supplement needs. The equivalent is valid for women who are pregnant and breastfeeding in light of expanded calorie and supplement needs,"

In case you're pregnant, you have to eat regularly and enough to help you and your child's wellbeing. The structure of intermittent fasting simply doesn't take into account that.

Are there options in contrast to intermittent fasting?

Unmistakably, intermittent fasting isn't for everybody. Be that as it may if the IF way of life isn't for you, is there an approach to receive all the rewards of intermittent fasting (like weight loss, expanded vitality, ideal fat burning, and better fixation) without putting yourself in danger?

The appropriate response is yes—with a guarantee to a sound, well-adjusted way of life. What's more, while that arrangement probably won't be as buzz-commendable as the intermittent fasting fever, it can surely be similarly as viable.
To add to your sound way of life, exercises are significant.

"A lot of what we think about nutrition doesn't have feature making request since it's exhausting. Eat more plants, pick heart solid fats, eat lean creature proteins (on the off chance that you need)— yet additionally incorporate plant proteins—centre around assortment, drink water, stay away from included sugars, limit ultra-prepared foods. We, as a whole, know these things. "The key is to make that method for gobbling one that makes up most of your eating regimen, most of the time, and for most of your life."

On the off chance that you have a condition that keeps you from jumping on board the intermittent fasting train, you can at present appreciate all the wellbeing boosting benefits. Roll out positive improvements to your eating regimen that you can focus on continuing in the long haul.

"Similarly, as with any eating routine, the one you can adhere to is the one that will have the most effect. Changing your deduction to outline wellbeing conduct as the one you'll have forever will positively affect how you approach any change,"

TIPS AND TRICKS TO IMPROVE THE RESULTS

TIPS AND TRICKS TO IMPROVE THE RESULT OF INTERMITTENT FASTING

How would you ensure you get fruitful intermittent fasting results? Follow these tips and deceives for powerful weight loss!

1. Get into the Right Mindset

2. Choose How You Want to Fast

3. Stick to the Routine however much as could reasonably be expected

4. Stay Hydrated

5. Exercise Portion Control

6. Eat the Right Kinds of Food

7. Sleep Well

Get the Intermittent Fasting Results You Seek with These 7 Tips

1. Get into the Right Mindset

Many individuals neglect to accomplish their intermittent fasting results since they couldn't set the correct mindset. They quit before they can even observe the progressions they need.

Otherwise called IF, intermittent fasting can't and ought not to be a one-time program. Truth be told, you must be reliable and make it part of your way of life.

You should, likewise be clear about your objectives. It is safe to say that you are doing intermittent fasting for weight loss, for instance?

These goals will assist you with setting benchmarks when you have to survey whether IF is working for you or not.

A few people may not be a contender for IF. These can incorporate kids or individuals beneath 18 years of age, pregnant women, and those with feeble safe frameworks.

Regardless of whether you're sound, you ought not to continue with IF without getting leeway from your primary care physician. You need to guarantee you're fit as a fiddle before you start this.

2. Pick How You Want to Fast

What is intermittent fasting? It's a patterned time of fasting, which can be calorie limitation or non-eating of food, and utilization of food. With this definition, we have various types of IFs:

•   Intermittent Fasting 16/8 Method—You fast for 16 hours and eat inside the 8-hour window.

•   Warrior Diet—You eat for just four hours and fast for the rest of the time.

•   Alternative Days—You fast every other day or on chose days of the week.

•   500-Calorie—You pick the days when you limit your entire day calorie admission to just 500.

•   12-Hour Fast—You eat for just 12 hours and fast the remainder of the day.

•   Skipping Meals—You abstain from eating one of the three major dinners. For the most part, it's breakfast.

In case you're a fledgeling, you might need in the first place a 12-hour fast and afterwards work your approach to 16:8, which numerous individuals do.

Note, however, fasting for longer periods can have wellbeing repercussions, for example, gallstone development. The hazard is higher among women, paying little mind to their weight.

Skipping breakfast may likewise not be perfect. This propensity will, in general, have a connect to atherosclerosis, a condition portrayed by the narrowing and solidifying of the supply routes.

On the off chance that you genuinely need to skip breakfast, you may substitute it with Rising Energy, which works like espresso yet without the jitter. It can give you the vitality you need until your first feast of the day.

3. Adhere to the Routine however much as could be expected

You're liked IF type just comes auxiliary to your promise to the daily schedule. However much as could be expected, you need to pick an intermittent fasting plan you can follow strictly.

These tips may support you:

- Make dinner your last supper so your rest can check toward the fasting time frame.

- Plan ahead for the exercises of the week. In the event that you hope to go to a birthday lunch on Friday, alter your fasting period the day preceding that.

- Keep yourself occupied, so you don't wind up speculation and getting food in the fast.

- Do you intend to work out? Do it after the fast, if conceivable.

4. Remain Hydrated

A man drinks water while climbing.

One of the fast effects of IF is hunger, and when you're eager, you are bound to imperil your intermittent fasting results.

To maintain a strategic distance from it, savour something between in the event that allows you to expend homegrown teas, espresso, and water during your fast.

You can even go for espresso options, which can help renew vitality, or a beverage utilizing Alkalizing Greens, a low-calorie mix that sustains your body with super greens.

5. Exercise Portion Control

Because you're doing the intermittent fasting diet doesn't mean you have the privilege to expend as much as you need during your non-fast period. This lone counterbalances the benefits of intermittent fasting.

You despite everything need to practice partition control, yet it might be troublesome when you can feel your stomach protesting. One of the methods is to pace your suppers, so you don't need to eat huge ones during your non-fast window.

In case you're on an 8-hour nourishing window, you may consider the accompanying timetable:

- First Hour—Eat your first ordinary dinner.

- Second Hour—Have a little tidbit.

- Third Hour—Eat your second last ordinary feast.

- The fifth Hour—Have another little tidbit.

- Seventh Hour—Eat your last ordinary feast.

Drink a lot of solid liquids between these suppers, and on the off chance that it helps, utilize a littler plate for better part control.

6. Eat the Right Kinds of Food

Eating the correct sorts of food is the ideal supplement to divide control. When IF leaves you wanting with regards to food, you may, in general, get microwavable suppers or head to the closest burger-and-fry shop.

You may likewise consider drinking improved refreshments in light of the fact that, all things considered, you trust you have to build your carbs.

All these won't give you the intermittent fasting results you need. Prepared foods, particularly ultra-handled foods, can leave you feeling much hungrier. More terrible, you're expanding your danger of metabolic conditions, including heftiness.
Here are a few hints for eating strongly:

•   Focus on foods with sound fats, for example, avocados and salmon.

•   Eat sound and lean proteins, for example, grass-sustained meat or chicken.

•   Stuff your plate with verdant greens.

•   Consume a few nuts as snacks.

•   Consider solid food swaps.

7. Rest soundly

A lady is resting in her bed.

You can likewise lose or not accomplish your ideal intermittent fasting results on the off chance that you need rest. Lack of sleep can prompt numerous issues, including the poor capacity to control hunger.

It can build the generation of a hormone called ghrelin, which animates the craving. It might likewise diminish the arrival of leptin, which should control it.

Absence of rest may likewise make you need to eat more treats and different types of desserts. This is on the grounds that it might enact endocannabinoid, a similar kind of lipid you animate when you take the pot.

Give yourself, at any rate, seven hours of rest. In case you're making some hard memories dozing, enhancements, for example, Relax and Unwind may help keep your resting designs ordinary.

This intermittent fasting guide carries you closer to the intermittent fasting results you need, yet just in case you're willing to buckle down for it. It's alright on the off chance that you flop every so often, as a great many people do.

What's basic is you refocus when you can, if you have your primary care physician's favouring and it's doing your body some great.

Here are different tips to assist you with fasting securely.

Continue Fasting Periods Short

There is no single method to fast; implying that the term of your fast is up to you.

Mainstream regimens include:

•   The 5:2 Pattern: Restrict your calorie admission for two days out of each week (500 calories for every day for women and 600 for men).

•   The 6:1 Pattern: This example is like the 5:2, yet there's just a single day of diminished calorie consumption rather than two.

•   "Eat Stop Eat": A 24-hour complete fast 1–2 times each week.

•   The 16:8 Pattern: This example includes just devouring food in an eight-hour window and fasting for 16 hours per day, each day of the week.

The greater part of these regimens instructs short fast periods concerning 8–24 hours. Notwithstanding, a few people decide to attempt any longer fasts of 48 and even as long as 72 hours.

Longer fast periods increment your danger of issues related to fasting. This incorporates drying out, touchiness, state of mind changes, swooning, hunger, an absence of vitality and being not able to centre The ideal approach to dodge these side effects is to adhere to shorter fasting times of as long as 24 hours — particularly when you're simply beginning.

In the event that you need to expand your fasting period to over 72 hours, you should look for medicinal supervision.

Longer times of fasting increment your danger of side effects, for example, lack of hydration, unsteadiness and blacking out. To diminish your hazard, keep your fasting periods short.

Eat a Small Amount on Fast Days

When all is said in done, fasting includes the evacuation of a few or all food and drink for a while.

In spite of the fact that you can expel food out and out on fast days, some fasting designs like the permit you to expend up to around 25% of your calorie prerequisites in a day.

In the event that you need to take a stab at fasting, limiting your calories so you despite everything eat modest quantities on your fast days might be a more secure choice than doing an all-out fast.

This methodology may help diminish a portion of the dangers related to fasting, for example, feeling weak, eager and unfocused.

Remain Hydrated

Mellow lack of hydration can bring about fatigue, dry mouth, thirst and cerebral pains — so it's imperative to drink enough liquid on a fast

Most wellbeing specialists suggest the 8x8 principle — eight 8-ounce glasses (just shy of 2 litres altogether) of liquid consistently — to remain hydrated.

Be that as it may, the genuine measure of liquid you need — albeit likely right now is very personal.

Since you get around 20–30% of the liquid your body needs from food, it's very simple to get dried out while on a fast

During fast, numerous individuals intend to drink 8.5–13 cups (2–3 litres) of water through the span of the day. In any case, your thirst should disclose to you when you have to drink more, so tune in to your body

As you meet a portion of your day by day liquid needs through food, you can get got dried out while fasting. To forestall this, tune in to your body and drink when parched.

Take Strolls or Meditate

Abstaining from eating on fast days can be troublesome, particularly on the off chance that you are feeling exhausted and hungry.

One approach to stay away from inadvertently breaking your fast is to keep occupied.

Exercises that may divert you from hunger — however, don't go through an excessive amount of vitality — incorporate strolling and ruminating.

In any case, any action that is quieting and not very strenuous would keep your psyche locked in. You could clean up, read a book or tune in to a digital recording.

Keeping occupied with low-force exercises, for example, strolling or reflecting, may make your fast days simpler.

Try not to Break Fasts With a Feast.

It very well may be enticing after a time of limitation to celebrate by eating an immense dinner.

Notwithstanding, breaking your fast with a gala could leave you feeling enlarged and tired.

Moreover, on the off chance that you need to shed pounds, devouring may hurt your long haul objectives by easing back down or stopping your weight loss.

Since your general calorie portion impacts your weight, expending over the top calories after a fast will diminish your calorie shortfall.

An ideal approach to break a fast is to keep eating typically and get once more into your normal eating schedule. On the off chance that you eat a strangely huge supper after your fast day, you may wind up feeling tired and enlarged. Take a stab at moving tenderly go into your typical food routine.

Quit Fasting If You Feel Unwell

During a fast, you may feel somewhat drained, eager and touchy — yet you ought to never feel unwell.

To protect yourself, particularly on the off chance that you are new to fasting, consider constraining your fast periods to 24 hours or less and keeping a bite close by in the event that you begin to feel blackout or sick.

On the off chance that you do turn out to be sick or are worried about your wellbeing, ensure you quit fasting straight away.

A few signs that you should stop your fast and look for therapeutic assistance incorporate tiredness or shortcoming that keeps you from doing day by day assignments, just as sudden sentiments of ailment and inconvenience.

You may feel somewhat worn out or bad-tempered during your fast, however in the event that you begin to feel unwell; you should quit fasting right away.

Eat Enough Protein

Numerous individuals begin fasting as an approach to attempt to get more fit.

In any case, being in a calorie shortage can make you lose muscle, notwithstanding fat.

One approach to limit your muscle loss while fasting is to guarantee you are eating enough protein when you eat

Furthermore, on the off chance that you are eating modest quantities on fast days, including some protein could offer different benefits, including managing your appetite.

A few investigations recommend that devouring around 30% of a feast's calories from protein can essentially diminish your craving.

Consequently, eating some protein on fast days could help balance a portion of fasting's side effects.

Having enough protein during your fast may help limit muscle loss and hold your hunger under control.

Eat Plenty of Whole Foods on Non-Fasting Days

A great many people who fast are attempting to improve their wellbeing.

Despite the fact that fasting includes avoiding food, it's as yet imperative to keep up a sound way of life on days when you are not fasting.

Sound weight control plans dependent on entire foods are connected to a wide scope of medical advantages, including a decreased danger of malignant growth, coronary illness and other interminable ailments.

You can ensure your eating routine stays solid by picking entire foods like meat, fish, eggs, vegetables, leafy foods when you eat.

Eating entire foods when you aren't fasting may improve your wellbeing and keep you well during a fast.

Consider Supplements

On the off chance that you fast routinely, you may pass up basic supplements.

This is on the grounds that are routinely eating less calories makes it harder to meet your nutritional needs.

Truth be told, individuals following weight loss abstains from food are bound to be lacking in various fundamental supplements like iron, calcium and nutrient B12

All things considered, the individuals who fast normally ought to consider taking a multivitamin for significant serenity and to help forestall lacks.

So, it's in every case best to get your supplements from entire foods.

Standard fasting may expand your danger of nutritional insufficiencies, particularly on the off chance that you are in a calorie shortfall. Hence, a few people decide to take a multivitamin.

Keep Exercise Mild

A few people find that they can keep up their normal exercise routine while fasting, However, in case you're new to fasting, it's ideal for holding any activity to a low power — particularly from the outset — so you can perceive how you oversee.

Low-force exercises could incorporate strolling, mellow yoga, delicate extending and housework.

In particular, tune in to your body and rest on the off chance that you battle to practice while fasting.

Numerous individuals figure out how to take an interest in their customary exercise routine on fast days. Nonetheless, when you're new to fasting, it's prescribed just to do gentle exercise to perceive how you feel.

•   Take note of how the body changes.

Turning 50 is an achievement worth celebrating. In any case, at 50, the body begins to change in manners, you might not have been anticipating. Here are, for the most part, the manners in which your body begins changing after 40.

•   You may turn out to be increasingly distracted.

Distraction turns out to be increasingly normal.

On the off chance that you find that you've strolled into a room and can't recollect why, or out of nowhere overlook the name of somebody near you for a concise moment, you are not the only one. Your memory's sharpness and feeling of comprehension can begin to diminish at only 50 years or more. After you turn 50, your memory starts to take a downturn. It was once figured this didn't occur until age 60. Yet, don't stress excessively — having a "senior minute" is normal and doesn't really mean you have any type of dementia.

You might be frustrated to see this.

• Your hair will begin dropping out.

You may see diminishing hair.

Research recommends that your hair will probably begin diminishing after 40. However, note that diminishing hair ordinarily relies upon hereditary qualities. Nonetheless, in the event that you notice some diminishing after 40, don't be frightened. It's totally ordinary to begin losing hair as you get more established. In addition, there are a few nutrients and medications you can use to advance hair development, for example, Viviscal or biotin supplements.

This will turn out to be increasingly normal.

• Grey hair will turn out to be increasingly normal

Obstinate greys may show up.

Besides some hair diminishing, you may see hair shading evolving, as well. Silver hairs are about unavoidable as you age, and they can show themselves as right on time as your 20s. Be that as it may, you may truly begin to see those greys after 50. The more established you get, the greyer you'll get, yet don't concern yourself a lot with it. You can generally colour your hair or attempt uncommon shampoos or conditioners to assist battle with offing the shading change.

• For women, hot flashes become progressively normal.

Hot flashes may begin as right on time as 50.

It's that time in your life when you may start to encounter your first hot flashes. And keeping in mind that the normal age for menopause is 51, you can get hot flashes as ahead of schedule as 10 years before menopause. In the event that you experience one, don't be astonished; however, it probably won't imply that menopause is around the bend. You could, in any case, have numerous years prior to that occurs.

• Sex may be more diligently than it used to be

Your sexual coexistence might be influenced after 50.

For the two people, sex may not be as simple as it once might have been. As you get more established, your hormone levels begin to decrease. This implies you may not be all set immediately. For men, you may need to investigate male upgrade drugs, for example, Viagra. Also, for women, dryness can happen, so you should converse with your primary care physician about the ideal approach to forestall that. Be that as it may, a couple of obstructions don't mean you can't even now appreciate closeness.

Furthermore, this may get a piece lower.

Your sex drive may become lower than it used to be

Your moxie might be lower.

In the event that you and your accomplice are experiencing difficulty with sex, it might cause a loss of charisma. Also, after 40, it's basic for the sex drive to fade away a piece. Stress is the main consideration that can add to low charisma, and in case you're worried at work (which is normal at this age), you may have to a lesser degree a craving to be intimate. Women are twice as liable to encounter low moxie contrasted with men, yet it despite everything that happens to people, particularly as you age.

Shedding the pounds gets more diligently.

It's progressively hard to get thinner.

Weight loss won't come as effectively.

As you age, your metabolism eases back down. Furthermore, age 50 is the point at which you may truly begin to see how much slower it is. The pounds become simpler to pick up and harder to shed. Counteraction recommends tips for getting more fit after 50: Focus on supplements, don't skip dinners and eat less calories yet more regularly. At the point when that metabolism begins to slow, eating huge suppers may mean putting on more weight than you'd like, yet it doesn't mean you can't lose it.

Next: You may see a couple of these.

You may see a few wrinkles.

Saturate to help maintain a strategic distance from wrinkles.

At the point when you're 50 or more established, your face doesn't have the equivalent solid shine it might have had when you were 20. That is on the grounds that the fat cushions in the face lessen, leaving the skin looking droopy. Additionally, the skin gets drier than it used to be, which can make wrinkles look progressively characterized. It's essential to maintain skin saturated in control to lessen the presence of wrinkles. A few specialists likewise suggest fillers, yet try to locate a dependable specialist who can do them accurately.

Next: Your resistance for this gets lower.

You can't drink as a lot of liquor as you once could

You can't drink like you used to.

There are a few reasons your capacity to deal with liquor might be influenced in your 50s. As you age, you will, in general beverage less much of the time, which brings down your resilience. Also, your liver isn't what it used to be, so utilizing the entirety of that liquor turns out to be progressively troublesome as you age. And afterwards, there's the likelihood that you might be taking a bigger number of prescriptions than you once did. Meds can prompt trouble in utilizing liquor, contingent upon the medication.

Next: These rates may increment.

You're bound to get certain malignancies.

People are at a more serious hazard for specific malignancies.

As you get more seasoned, the wellbeing dangers become increasingly genuine. When you hit 50, certain diseases have a more noteworthy possibility of showing up. Bosom malignancy hazard increments once you turn 50, so you ought to get yearly mammograms to ensure everything looks great. Additionally, most instances of disease are analyzed in individuals more than 50. However, when you turn 50, you might need to converse with your primary care physician about what's in store not far off, for example, testing for colon and prostate tumours.

Next: Can you rehash that?

You may see the primary indications of hearing loss.

You may see the main indications of hearing loss.

It might appear as though an issue you don't have to stress over for another 20 or 30 years; however, hearing loss can begin to create as ahead of schedule as your 50s. It depends on how much strain your ears dealt with when you were more youthful. On the off chance that you went to shows regularly and were continually impacting music, you may see a hearing loss at a previous age than somebody who didn't tune in to a lot of uproarious music. In any case, it's normal to get yourself somewhat harder of hearing in your 50s.

Next: This may fall somewhat askew.

Your rest cycle may change.

Your rest cycle may change. | Povozniuk/iStock/Getty Images

As you get more established, your brain effectiveness decays. Furthermore, this can influence your rest design. At the point when you age, the brain delivers less melatonin, which can make falling and staying unconscious troublesome. You may end up nodding off on the lounge chair all the more frequently or awakening in the night. And keep in mind that genuine rest issues don't ordinarily begin until your 50s or 60s, converse with your primary care physician on the off chance that you notice any adjustments in your 50s since it could be an indication of rest trouble not far off.

Next: The odds of this will diminish.

Your odds of having kids — for females — diminishes.

Female richness decline.

The richness in the two sexual orientations diminishes after 50. Lady has a more noteworthy possibility of having an unnatural birth cycle. Women more than 50 are half as liable to get pregnant or have a solid infant than they were before age 32. Also, at age 30, women have a 20% possibility of getting pregnant in a given month. By age 50, it's just 3%.

Next: This is a typical issue in women more than 50.

Your bladder could become 'cracked.'

A cracked bladder turns out to be progressively normal after 50

For some women, more than 50, bladder incontinence is normal. As indicated by an examination done on women between the ages of 42 and 64, over 68% confessed to having bladder incontinence in any event once every month. The vast majority partner the bladder spillage with menopause; however, there is no proof the two are connected. Crumbling of specific muscles from labour may likewise add to the spillage.

Next: Your teeth will improve right now.

Your teeth become less delicate.

Your teeth become less delicate.

At the point when you hit your 50s, your teeth produce more dentin than they once did. This implies in the event that you've battled with touchy teeth for an incredible majority, and there is uplifting news: More dentin implies your teeth will feel less delicate. It couldn't be any more obvious. A few things improve age. Be that as it may, it's imperative to get dental exams in light of the fact that with less affectability comes less information on when something might not be right with your teeth.

TIPS AND TRICKS ON WALKING EVERYDAY TO INCREASE FAT BURNING

- Why you ought to stroll to shed pounds.

Strolling requires little in the method for hardware, it very well may be accomplished pretty much anyplace, and it's more averse to stretch the joints in the manner that running can.

Yet, in light of the fact that strolling upstanding is a simple, common route for people to consume vitality from the food we eat, it doesn't imply that we can't figure out how to improve—and increment the tummy consume.

By following the tips underneath, you'll figure out how strolling to get more fit is a low-sway approach to arrive at your body objectives.

Strolling tips before you go out.

1.   Choose the correct shoes. The main "gear" important for strolling (except if it's on the sea shore) are shoes and chances are you have a couple reasonable for the activity as of now. "Strolling shoes" have adaptable soles and solid heel counters to forestall side-to-side movement. Typical level surfaces just require low-obeyed shoes that are agreeable, padded and lightweight.

2.   Devise an extraordinary strolling playlist. Prior to you even consider binding up your tennis shoes, think about the tunes you need to hear as you make progress towards a fitter you. Having an incredible soundtrack to your walk will inspire you to push more diligently and go more remote and best of all, you most likely won't see the additional exertion that you wind up placing in. Search for tunes that are between 75 to 130 BPM—these rhythms will assist you with synchronizing your swagger to the beat.

3.   Know your course. It's acceptable to have an away from of where you'll be strolling on some random day. You'll feel great and certain recognizing what's in store as you walk and not burn through any strolling time making sense of a course on the fly. Attempt and devise a bunch of courses that change long, evaluation, and landscape. Only two or three-course alternatives can forestall your new stomach shooting propensity from getting monotonous.

4.   Find a mobile pal. Having a solid care group is crucial to accomplishing and keeping up weight loss achievement, with the individuals who are a piece of a social, encouraging group of people losing more weight than their independent partners.

5.   Find that strolling amigo diverting. It's a big deal: certified chuckling may cause a 10–20 per cent expansion in basal vitality consumption and resting heart-rate, That implies a 10 brief laugh-fest could consume 40 to 170 calories.

6.   Be arranged for climate conditions. We don't all live in San Diego, which implies that we need to manage a powerful atmosphere. Try not to let a run of blistering, chilly, wet, breezy or frosty climate keep you from strolling off your paunch. Get yourself kitted out with the correct attire for the sorts of climate your region can get in a given year. During a warmth wave, stroll

before the sun gets excessively high in the sky, during a frosty spell, do the inverse. A reasonable climate walker in Seattle or Fargo is going to pass up a great deal of tummy impacting openings.

7.Keep tabs on your steps. Some medical coverage organizations currently offer budgetary motivating forces for individuals who can clock up a specific number of steps in a day. That is on the grounds that they realize that strolling is an incredible method to fight off weight and ailment. There's no perfect number with regards to what number of day by day steps is perfect; however, Japanese wellbeing authorities exhort 10,000 stages as an objective. There's just a single method to discover what number of steps you're timing up: get a pedometer. They're generally modest and could wind up persuading you to shed a few pounds.

8.   Keep a mobile diary. Keeping a diary been appeared to build the viability of a mobile program by 47 per cent, Keep track of the days that you played out your strolling schedule, the hour of day or night that you played out your strolling schedule, the separation and time to finish each strolling everyday practice, the course wherein you played out your strolling schedule and your week after week weight.

9.   Walk-in sunshine to eat less. Go get a portion of that daylight or even sunshine on your walk. Why? Indeed, Sleep-denied grown-ups who were presented to diminish the light in the wake of waking had lower centralizations of the totality hormone leptin while those in blue light (the sort from vitality proficient bulbs) had higher leptin levels. By giving some light access to your life, you'll get some life into your weight-loss objectives as you walk toward a slimmer, more beneficial future.

The most effective method to stroll for weight loss.

1.   Hit the blocks before breakfast. The best technique for bringing body fat rate is down to get your walk not long after subsequent to awakening. "Your body is as of now in a calorie deficiency, and it will touch off your body's fat-burning capacity," "Glycogen levels are exhausted during rest, so your body will use body fat as a vitality source."

2.   Walk energetically. Walk like you're at the air terminal and you've cut it close for leaving flight. In case you're 150 pounds strolling energetically (around 3.5 miles every hour) will consume around 300 calories at regular intervals. On the off chance that you can fit shortly of lively strolling on a level surface each day, you'll have consumed off 1,050 calories before the week's over. This kind of week after week calorie consumption ensures against coronary illness and obviously, you'll presumably begin seeing that you look and feel changed soon.

3.   But additionally, fluctuate your strolling pace. Strolling at different velocities can wreck to 20 per cent more calories contrasted with keeping up a relentless pace Is one of the first to gauge the metabolic expense, or calories consumed, of changing strolling speeds. While strolling energetically for 30 minutes is a good thought, attempt and work in no time flat in which you fasten and decelerate your lively walk.

4.   Swing your arms. It couldn't be any more obvious, energetic arm siphoning not just speeds your pace, it additionally gives a decent chest area exercise. Furthermore: an arm swinging strolling style will make you consume 5 to 10 per cent more calories. Twist your arms at 90 degrees and siphon from the shoulder. Swing them normally, as though you're going after your wallet in your back pocket. On the swing forward, your wrist ought to be close to the focal point of your chest.

The most effective method to help weight loss while strolling.

1.   Go faster the correct way. In the event that you need to expand your strolling pace, there are two different ways you can do it. You can take long walks, or you can fastly walk. It's smarter to do them later on the grounds that protracting your walk can expand strain on your feet and legs.

2.   Vary the territory. Just as changing your speed, an extraordinary method to consume more paunch fat is to switch up the surface you're strolling on. Obviously, strolling on grass or rock consumes a bigger number of calories than strolling on a track while strolling on delicate sand increments caloric consumption by just about 50 per cent, given that you can keep your pace the equivalent.

3.   Add high-force strolls to your daily practice. Do in any event 20 minutes of high-force strolling on 3 nonconsecutive days of the week as you'll consume progressively fat during and after these cardio-escalated exercises. On alternate days, do direct force wellness action for around 30 minutes for every session.

4.   Walk tough. Strolling energetically up a short slope is an extraordinary case of interim preparing when mixed with level landscape strolling. Your leg muscles with thank you on the off chance that you slender forward somewhat when strolling tough and your knees will be much increasingly appreciative on the off chance that you moderate your pace, twist your legs marginally and make shorter strides when you plunge those slopes.

5.   Ski the boulevards. Upgrade your chest area exercise by utilizing lightweight, elastic tipped trekking shafts. On the off chance that you've cross-country skiing ever, you'll know the development. In the event that you haven't, it goes this way: Step forward with the left foot as the correct arm with the post approaches and is planted on the ground, about even with the impact point of the left foot. Strolling with posts while lessening the weight on your knees while working the muscles of your chest and arms just as certain abs.

6.   Use hand weights. Hand weights can help your caloric use, yet they may adjust your arm swing and therefore lead to muscle irritation or even damage. They're by and large not prescribed for individuals with hypertension or coronary illness. On the off chance that you need to utilize them, start with one-pound weights and increment the weight steadily. The weights shouldn't mean in excess of 10 per cent of your body weight. Lower leg weights are not suggested, as they increment the possibility of damage.

7.   Try in reverse or "retro" strolling. Strolling in reverse uses the leg muscles uniquely in contrast to strolling advance and can be an incredible method for restoring from knee damage. Retro strolling is most secure on a treadmill, yet an abandoned running track would be similarly as appropriate. On the off chance that you have neither of those settings accessible to you, stroll outside—away from traffic, trees, potholes, and so forth.— with a spotter. Indeed, even a moderate pace (2 mph) gives genuinely exceptional training. To maintain a strategic distance from muscle irritation, start gradually: don't attempt to walk in reverse in excess of a quarter mile the primary week.

Tips for post-walk.

1.   Drink green tea subsequent to strolling. This implies green tea can likewise assist you with recuperating faster after an energetic walk. Individuals who matched drinking a games refreshment with what might be compared to four to five cups of green tea with a 30-minute run three times each week for about two months expanded their capacity to consume fat during exercise just as while they were stationary.

2.   Or beverage plain water. Fast weight loss doesn't get simpler than this: Simply drinking more water may build the rate at which solid individuals consume calories, After drinking roughly 17 ounces of water (around 2 tall glasses) metabolic rates expanded by 30 per cent.

3.   Just as long as you do without sports drinks. Ever observe somebody expending a Gatorade or Vitaminwater while strolling? Except if they're strolling up a sharp grade in a rush, they're treating it terribly. "Numerous individuals feel they need these sugar-thick beverages after shorter or less exceptional exercises," "in all actuality, these beverages frequently have a bigger number of calories in them than what's really being singed off." Her recommendation isn't to expend such beverages except if you work out with a raised pulse for at any rate 60 minutes. "Generally these beverages are required because of the danger of parchedness," however alerts that in case you're strolling in gentle temperatures or for not exactly 60 minutes, they're to a great extent superfluous. Besides, those sugary beverages are horrendous nutrition for sprinters and walkers, at any rate!

4.   Snack on almonds. A low-calorie diet that is wealthy in almonds could assist increment with weighting loss. Not exclusively do the great monounsaturated fats in almonds affect insulin levels, yet in addition give health food nuts a full inclination, implying that they are more averse to indulge. To expedite a little pack of almonds, your walk in the event that you start to feel hungry.

5.   Make your walk a piece of your life. From the start, anything new can be hard to continue doing, just in light of the fact that it's not part of your daily schedule yet. When it turns into a propensity, it will end up being a piece of your everyday stream. Recall that inspiration is the thing that kicks you off and propensities are what prop you up.

6.	Do progressively accidental strolling, as well. Strolling for weight loss is a certain something. However, strolling has different benefits, also. Reward stomach fat burning open doors anticipate you on the off chance that you can leave the vehicle at home, take the stairs rather than lifts and elevators or on the off chance that you can walk the mile or two to a companion or relative's home. On the off chance that you take mass travel to work, stroll to a transport or train stop somewhat further along the course.

7.	Don't starve yourself after your walk. "Post-exercise nutrition is critical to any wellness objectives," says Santoro, who keeps up that pre-and post-exercise nutrition is the two most significant suppers of your day. It's critical to refuel your body following an exercise or lively walk since it renews glycogen levels, decline protein breakdown, and increment protein union and the capacity to fabricate muscle.

8.	But don't eat more than your walk consumed. An incredible 70 to 75 per cent of the calories we exhaust every day is required for our "basal metabolic functions:" Everything from keeping your heart thumping to causing your fingernails to develop. At the point when we apply a great deal of additional vitality in the rec centre, our bodies get out for more fuel with food cravings and a thundering gut. Now, individuals will, in general, undermine their endeavours with foods that really make them hungrier or unnecessary measure of food "When to work out actuated craving sets in, just increment your calorie admission up to 20 to 30 per cent of what your calorie tracker says you consumed," she says.

9.	Pair your strolling with some opposition preparing. In any event, when you're very still, your body is continually burning calories. Truth be told, 75 per cent of the calories that you consume every day are being spent simply keeping you alive. "Resting metabolic rate" is a lot higher in individuals with more muscle, in light of the fact that each pound of muscle utilizes around 6 calories per day just to continue itself. In the event that you can pack on only five pounds of muscle and support it, you'll consume what might be compared to three pounds of fat through the span of a year. Pair that additional sturdiness with 30 minutes of lively strolling once every day, and you'll begin eliminating your additional fat stores right away.

10.	Walk to de-stress. Strolling energetically or running truly calms you somewhere near starting nerve cells in the brain that loosen up the faculties. What's more, that is uplifting news for your weight loss objectives. It's just plain obvious; stress can really make the body process food all the more gradually. The food we hunger for when we're worried will, in general, be fatty and loaded with sugar. Analysts state that the blend of high-cal desires and a pressure-actuated, snail-paced metabolic rate can bring about huge weight gain. Thus, by strolling to shed pounds and decrease pressure, you won't be pressure eating to such an extent: it's a success win.

TIPS AND TRICKS ON INTERMITTENT FASTING TO IMPROVE DIGESTION

The 11 Best Ways to Improve Your Digestion Naturally

Everybody encounters infrequent stomach-related side effects, for example, annoyed stomach, gas, acid reflux, sickness, obstruction or lose bowels.

In any case, when these side effects happen much of the time, they can make significant interruptions your life.

Luckily, diet and way of life changes can positively affect your gut wellbeing.

Here are 11 proof-based approaches to improve your absorption normally.

1. Eat Real Food

The run of the mill Western eating routine — high in refined carbs, immersed fat and food added substances — has been connected to an expanded danger of creating stomach related disarranges.

Food added substances, including glucose, salt and different synthetic substances, have been recommended to add to expanded gut irritation, prompting a condition called the flawed gut.

Trans fats are found in many prepared foods. They're notable for their negative effects on heart wellbeing however have likewise been related with an expanded danger of creating ulcerative colitis, an incendiary entrail malady.

In addition, prepared foods like low-calorie beverages and frozen yoghurts frequently contain fake sugars, which may mess stomach related up.

Eating 50 grams of the fake sugar xylitol prompted swelling and looseness of the bowels in 70% of individuals, while 75 grams of the sugar erythritol caused similar side effects in 60% of individuals.

Fake sugars may expand your number of destructive gut microorganisms.

Gut microscopic organisms awkward nature have been connected to fractious gut disorder (IBS) and crabby entrail sicknesses like ulcerative colitis and Crohn's infection.

Luckily, logical proof recommends that eats less high in supplements secure against stomach related illnesses.

In this way, eating an eating routine dependent on entire foods and constraining the admission of prepared foods might be best for ideal absorption.

Diets high in handled foods have been connected to a higher danger of stomach related disarranges. Eating an eating routine low in food added substances, trans fats and counterfeit sugars may improve your absorption and secure against stomach related sicknesses.

2. Get Plenty of Fiber

It's regular information that fibre is helpful for acceptable absorption.

Dissolvable fibre retains water and encourages add mass to your stool. Insoluble fibre acts like a goliath toothbrush, helping your stomach related tract keep everything moving along.

Solvent fibre is found in oat wheat, vegetables, nuts and seeds, while vegetables, entire grains and wheat grain are acceptable wellsprings of insoluble fibre.

A high-fibre diet has been connected to a decreased danger of stomach related conditions, including ulcers, reflux, haemorrhoids, diverticulitis and IBS.

Prebiotics are another sort of fibre that feed your sound gut microbes. Diets high right has now been appeared to lessen the danger of incendiary entrail conditions.

Prebiotics are found in numerous organic products, vegetables and grains.

A high-fibre diet advances ordinary solid discharges and may ensure against numerous stomach related clutters. Three basic types of fibre are solvent and insoluble fibre, just as prebiotics.

3. Add Healthy Fats to Your Diet

Great assimilation may require eating enough fat. Fat causes you feel fulfilled after dinner and is frequently required for appropriate supplement assimilation.

Moreover, considers have indicated that omega-3 fatty acids may diminish your danger of creating incendiary inside ailments like ulcerative colitis.

Foods high in helpful omega-3 fatty acids incorporate flaxseeds, chia seeds, nuts (particularly pecans), just as fatty fish like salmon, mackerel and sardines.

Satisfactory fat admission improves the assimilation of some fat-solvent supplements. Furthermore, omega-3 fatty acids decrease aggravation, which may forestall provocative inside sicknesses.

4. Remain hydrated

Low liquid admission is a typical reason for the blockage. Specialists suggest drinking 50–66 ounces (1.5–2 litres) of non-juiced liquids every day to forestall stoppage. Be that as it may, you may require more on the off chance that you live in a warm atmosphere or exercise strenuously.

Notwithstanding water, you can likewise meet your liquid admission with homegrown teas and other non-juiced drinks, for example, seltzer water.

Another approach to help meet your liquid admission needs is to incorporate leafy foods that are high in water, for example, cucumber, zucchini, celery, tomatoes, melons, strawberries, grapefruit and peaches.

Inadequate liquid admission is a typical reason for the stoppage. Increment your water consumption by drinking non-stimulated refreshments and eating leafy foods that have high water content.

5. Deal with Your Stress

Stress can unleash devastation on your stomach related framework.

It has been related with stomach ulcers, looseness of the bowels, stoppage and IBS.

Stress hormones legitimately influence your assimilation. At the point when your body is in battle or-flight mode, it figures you don't have the opportunity to rest and process. During times of pressure, blood and vitality are occupied away from your stomach related framework.

Moreover, your gut and brain are unpredictably associated — what influences your brain may likewise affect your assimilation.

Stress the board, reflection and unwinding preparing have all been appeared to improve side effects in individuals with IBS.

Intellectual conduct treatment, needle therapy and yoga have improved stomach related manifestations.

Accordingly, joining pressure the executives' methods, for example, profound stomach breathing, reflection or yoga, may improve your mindset as well as your processing.

Stress contrarily impacts your processing and has been connected to IBS, ulcers, obstruction and looseness of the bowels. Diminishing pressure can improve stomach-related side effects.

6. Eat Mindfully

It's anything but difficult to eat a lot of too rapidly in case you're not focusing, which can prompt swelling, gas and heartburn.

Careful eating is the act of focusing on all parts of your food and the way toward eating.

Studies have indicated that care may lessen stomach-related side effects in individuals with ulcerative colitis and IBS.

To eat carefully:

- Eat gradually.

- Focus on your food by killing your TV and taking care of your telephone.

- Notice how your food looks on your plate and how it smells.

- Select each chomp of food intentionally.

- Pay consideration regarding the surface, temperature and taste of your food.

Eating gradually and carefully and focusing on each part of your food, for example, surface, temperature and taste, may help forestall regular stomach related problems, for example, acid reflux, swelling and gas.

7. Bite Your Food

Assimilation begins in your mouth. Your teeth separate the food into little pieces with the goal that the chemicals in your stomach related tract are better ready to separate it.

Poor biting has been connected to diminished supplement assimilation.

At the point when you bite your food altogether, your stomach needs to do less work to transform the strong food into the fluid blend that enters your small digestive tract.

Biting produces spit, and the more you bite, the more salivation is made. Spit helps start the stomach related procedure in your mouth by separating a portion of the carbs and fats in your supper.

In your stomach, spit goes about as a liquid, which is blended in with the strong food, so it easily goes into your digestive organs.

Biting your food completely guarantees that you have a lot of spit for processing. This may help forestall side effects, for example, acid reflux and indigestion.

Additionally, the demonstration of biting has even been appeared to lessen pressure, which may likewise improve processing.

Biting food completely separates it with the goal that it very well may be processed all the more effectively. The demonstration additionally creates spit, which is required for the legitimate blending of food in your stomach.

8. Get Going

Normal exercise is perhaps the ideal approaches to improve your absorption.

Exercise and gravity assist food with going through your stomach related framework. In this way, going for a stroll after dinner may help your body in moving things along.

Moderate exercise, for example, cycling and running, expanded gut travel time by almost 30%

Day by day practice routine including 30 minutes of strolling altogether improved indications

Furthermore, examines propose that activity may lessen manifestations of provocative gut infections because of anti-incendiary effects, for example, diminishing fiery mixes in your body.

Exercise may improve your assimilation and diminish the manifestations of blockage. It can likewise help lessen irritation, which might be valuable in forestalling incendiary gut conditions.

9. Slow Down and Listen to Your Body

At the point when you're not focusing on your appetite and completion prompts, it's anything but difficult to indulge and encounter gas, swelling and heartburn.

It's a familiar way of thinking that it takes 20 minutes for your brain to understand that your stomach is full.

While there's not a great deal of hard science to back up this case, it takes time for hormones discharged by your stomach because of food to arrive at your brain.

In this way, setting aside the effort to eat gradually and focus on how full you're getting is one approach to forestall normal stomach related issues.

Also, passionate eating adversely impacts your assimilation. In one investigation, individuals who ate when they were restless experienced more elevated levels of heartburn and swelling.

Setting aside the effort to unwind before dinner may improve your stomach-related side effects.

Not focusing on your craving and totality signs and eating when you're enthusiastic or on edge can contrarily affect assimilation. Setting aside some effort to unwind and focus on your body's prompts may help diminish stomach related indications after a feast.

10. Jettison Bad Habits

You realize that negative behaviour patterns, for example, smoking, drinking a lot of liquor and eating late around evening time aren't incredible for your general wellbeing.

Furthermore, truth be told, they may likewise be answerable for some basic stomach related problems.

✓ Smoking

Smoking almost pairs the danger of creating indigestion. Besides, considers have indicated that stopping smoking improves these manifestations.

This unfortunate propensity has additionally been related to stomach ulcers, expanded medical procedures in individuals with ulcerative colitis and gastrointestinal diseases.

In the event that you have stomach related problems and smoke cigarettes, remember that stopping might be advantageous.

✓ Liquor

Liquor can expand corrosive generation in your stomach and may prompt indigestion, heartburn and stomach ulcers.

Exorbitant liquor utilization has been connected to seeping in the gastrointestinal tract.

Liquor has likewise been related with fiery inside sicknesses, flawed gut and hurtful changes in gut microorganisms.

Lessening your utilization of liquor may support your processing.

✓ Late-Night Eating

Eating late around evening time and afterwards resting to rest can prompt acid reflux and heartburn.

Your body needs time to process, and gravity helps keep the food you eat moving the correct way.

Also, when you rest, the substance of your stomach may ascend and cause indigestion. Resting in the wake of eating is unequivocally connected with an expansion in reflux indications.

On the off chance that you experience stomach related problems at sleep time, take a stab at holding up three to four hours subsequent to eating before heading to sleep, to give the food time to move from your stomach to your small digestive tract.

Unfortunate propensities, for example, smoking, drinking an excessive amount of liquor and eating late around evening time can cause stomach related problems. To improve assimilation, attempt to maintain a strategic distance from these damaging propensities.

11. Join Gut-Supporting Nutrients

Certain supplements may help bolster your stomach related tract.

Probiotics

Probiotics are gainful microscopic organisms that may improve stomach related wellbeing when taken as enhancements.

These sound microbes aid processing by separating toxic strands that can result in any case cause gas and swelling.

Studies have indicated that probiotics may improve side effects of swelling, gas and agony in individuals with IBS.

In addition, they may improve side effects of blockage and loose bowels.

Probiotics are found in aged foods, for example, sauerkraut, kimchi and miso, just as yoghurts that have live and dynamic societies.

They're likewise accessible in container structure. A decent broad probiotic supplement will contain a blend of strains including Lactobacillus and Bifidobacterium.

Glutamine

Glutamine is an amino corrosive that supports gut wellbeing. It has been appeared to lessen intestinal porousness (cracked gut) in individuals who are fundamentally sick.

You can expand your glutamine levels by eating foods, for example, turkey, soybeans, eggs and almonds.

Glutamine can likewise be taken in supplement structure, yet converse with your social insurance specialist first to guarantee that it's a suitable treatment system for you.

Zinc

Zinc is a mineral that is basic for a sound gut, and a lack can prompt different gastrointestinal issue.

Enhancing with zinc has been demonstrated to be useful in treating loose bowels, colitis, broken gut and other stomach related problems.

The suggested every day admission (RDI) for zinc is 8 mg for women and 11 mg for men.

Foods high in zinc incorporate shellfish, meat and sunflower seeds.

Certain supplements are fundamental for a sound stomach related tract. Guaranteeing that your body gets enough probiotics, glutamine and zinc may improve your assimilation.

Straightforward eating routine and way of life changes may help improve your assimilation on the off chance that you experience periodic, visit or constant stomach related manifestations.

Eating an entire foods diet high in fibre, sound fat and supplements is the initial move toward great absorption.

Practices, for example, careful eating, stress decrease and exercise can likewise be valuable.

At long last, discarding negative behaviour patterns that may influence your absorption —, for example, smoking, drinking an excess of liquor and late-evening eating — may help alleviate indications also.

TIPS AND TRICKS TO IMPROVE SLEEP IN INTERMITTENT FASTING

Demonstrated Tips to Sleep Better at Night for women

A decent night's rest is similarly as significant as customary exercise and a sound eating routine.

Poor rest has fast negative effects on your hormones, practice execution and brain work. It can likewise cause weight addition and increment ailment chance in the two grown-ups and youngsters.

Conversely, great rest can assist you with eating less, practice better and be more advantageous.

In the course of recent decades, both rest quality and quantity has declined. Indeed, numerous individuals routinely get poor rest.

On the off chance that you need to improve your wellbeing or get thinner, at that point, getting a decent night's rest is one of the most significant things you can do.

Here are 17 proof-based tips to rest better around evening time.

1. Increment Bright Light Exposure during the Day

Your body makes some common memories keeping clock known as your circadian mood.

It influences your brain, body and hormones, helping you remain wakeful and advising your body when it's an ideal opportunity to rest.

Regular daylight or splendid light during the day helps keep your circadian cadence solid. This improves daytime vitality, just as evening time rest quality and length.

In individuals with a sleeping disorder, daytime splendid light presentation improved rest quality and span. It likewise diminished the time it took to nod off by 83%.

Two hours of splendid light presentation during the day expanded the measure of rest by two hours and rest proficiency by 80%.

Individuals with extreme rest issues, day by daylight introduction will in all probability assist you with a night on the off chance that you experience normal rest.

Take a stab at getting day by day daylight introduction or — if this isn't handy — put resources into a counterfeit brilliant light gadget or bulbs.

Every day daylight or fake brilliant light can improve rest quality and term, particularly on the off chance that you have serious rest issues or a sleeping disorder.

2. Diminish Blue Light Exposure in the Evening

Introduction to light during the day is gainful. However, evening time light presentation has the contrary impact.

Once more, this is because of its effect on your circadian beat, fooling your brain into speculation it is still daytime. This diminishes hormones like melatonin, which assist you with unwinding and get profound rest.

Blue light — which electronic gadgets like cell phones and PCs emanate in enormous sums — is the most exceedingly terrible right now.

There are a few well-known techniques you can use to diminish evening blue light presentation. These include:

• Wear glasses that square blue light.

• Download an application, for example, f.lux to square blue light on your PC or PC.

• Install an application that squares blue light on your cell phone. These are accessible for both iPhones and Android models.

• Stop sitting in front of the TV and mood killer any splendid lights two hours before going to bed.

Blue light fools your body into believing it's daytime. There are a few different ways you can diminish blue light introduction at night.

3. Try not to Consume Caffeine Late in the Day

In any case, when expended late in the day, espresso invigorates your sensory system and may prevent your body from normally unwinding around evening time.

Devouring caffeine as long as six hours before bed altogether declined rest quality

Caffeine can remain raised in your blood for 6–8 hours. In this manner, drinking a lot of espresso after 3–4 p.m. isn't prescribed — particularly in the event that you are delicate to caffeine or experience difficulty resting.

In the event that you do need some espresso in the late evening or night, stay with decaffeinated espresso.

Caffeine can essentially intensify rest quality, particularly on the off chance that you drink huge sums in the late evening or night.

4. Decrease Irregular or Long Daytime Naps

While short force snoozes are helpful, long or unpredictable resting during the day can adversely influence your rest.

Resting in the daytime can befuddle your inside clock, implying that you may battle to rest around evening time.

Truth be told, in one investigation, members wound up being sleepier during the day subsequent to taking daytime snoozes.

While resting for 30 minutes or less can upgrade daytime brain work, longer snoozes can adversely influence wellbeing and rest quality.

Nonetheless, a few investigations exhibit that the individuals who are accustomed to taking customary daytime snoozes don't encounter poor rest quality or disturbed rest around evening time.

On the off chance that you take standard daytime snoozes and rest soundly, you shouldn't need to stress. The effects of snoozing rely upon the person.

Long daytime may impede rest quality. In the event that you experience difficulty dozing around evening time, quit resting or abbreviate your snoozes.

5. Attempt to Sleep and Wake at Consistent Times

Your body's circadian cadence functions on a set circle, adjusting itself to dawn and dusk.

Being steady with your rest and waking occasions can help long haul rest quality One investigation noticed that members who had unpredictable dozing designs and hit the sack late on the ends of the week revealed poor rest.

Unpredictable rest examples can modify your circadian mood and levels of melatonin, which signal your brain to rest.

On the off chance that you battle with rest, attempt to start awakening and heading to sleep at comparable occasions. Following a little while, you may not require an alert.

Attempt to get into a normal rest/wake cycle — particularly on the ends of the week. On the off chance that conceivable, attempt to wake up normally at a comparative time each day.

6. Take a Melatonin Supplement

Melatonin is a key rest hormone that advises your brain when it's a great opportunity to unwind and go to bed.

Melatonin supplements are an amazingly well-known tranquillizer.

Frequently used to treat a sleeping disorder, melatonin might be probably the most effortless approaches to nod off faster.

2 mg of melatonin before bed improved rest quality and vitality the following day and helped individuals nod off faster. In another investigation, half of the gathering nodded off faster and had a 15% improvement in rest quality.

Also, no withdrawal effects were accounted for in both of the above investigations.

Melatonin is additionally valuable when making a trip and acclimating to another time zone, as it enables your body's circadian mood to come back to typical.

In certain nations, you need a solution for melatonin. In others, melatonin is generally accessible in stores or on the web. Take around 1–5 mg 30–an hour prior to bed.

Start with a low portion to evaluate your resilience, and afterwards increment it gradually varying. Since melatonin may modify brain science, it is exhorted that you check with a therapeutic expert before use.

You ought to likewise talk with a medicinal services supplier in case you're contemplating utilizing melatonin as a tranquillizer for your youngster, as long haul utilization of this enhancement in kids has not been all around examined.

A melatonin supplement is a simple method to improve rest quality and nod off faster. Take 1–5 mg around 30–an hour prior to making a beeline for bed.

7. Consider These Other Supplements

A few enhancements can instigate unwinding and help you rest, including:

•   Ginkgo biloba: A characteristic herb with numerous benefits, it might help in rest, unwinding and stress decrease; however, the proof is restricted. Take 250 mg 30–an hour prior to bed.

•   Glycine: A couple of studies show that 3 grams of the corrosive amino glycine can improve rest quality

•   Valerian root: Several examinations propose that valerian can assist you with nodding off and improve rest quality. Take 500 mg before bed Magnesium: Responsible for more than 600 responses inside your body, magnesium can improve unwinding and upgrade rest quality.

•   L-theanine: An amino corrosive, l-theanine can improve unwinding and rest. Take 100–200 mg before bed.

•   Lavender: An amazing herb with numerous medical advantages, lavender can incite a quieting and stationary impact to improve rest. Take 80–160 mg containing 25–46% linalool.

Try just to attempt these enhancements each in turn. While they are no enchantment projectile for rest issues, they can be valuable when joined with other common dozing techniques.

A few enhancements, including lavender and magnesium, can help with unwinding and rest quality when joined with different systems.

8. Try not to Drink Alcohol

Bringing down two or three beverages around evening time can contrarily influence your rest and hormones.

Liquor is known to cause or expand the indications of rest apnea, wheezing and disturbed rest designs.

It additionally adjusts evening time melatonin generation, which assumes a key job in your body's circadian musicality.

Another investigation found that liquor utilization around evening time diminished the characteristic evening time rises in human development hormone (HGH), which assumes a job in your circadian beat and has numerous other key functions.

Dodge liquor before bed, as it can lessen evening time melatonin generation and lead to disturbed rest designs.

9. Upgrade Your Bedroom Environment

Numerous individuals accept that the room condition and its arrangement are key factors in getting a decent night's rest.

These variables incorporate temperature, clamour, outside lights and furniture course of action.

Various investigations call attention to that outside commotion, frequently from traffic, can cause poor rest and long haul medical problems.

In one examination on the room condition of women, around 50% of members saw improved rest quality when commotion and light lessened.

To enhance your room condition, attempt to limit outer clamour, light and fake lights from gadgets like morning timers. Ensure your room is a peaceful, unwinding, perfect and pleasant spot.

Improve your room condition by killing outside light and clamour to show signs of improvement rest.

10. Set Your Bedroom Temperature

Body and room temperature can likewise significantly affect rest quality.

As you may have encountered throughout the late spring or in hot areas, it tends to be extremely difficult to get a decent night's rest when it's excessively warm.

One investigation found that room temperature influenced rest quality more than outer clamour.

Different investigations uncover that expanded body and room temperature can diminish rest quality and increment attentiveness.

Around 70°F (20°C) is by all accounts an agreeable temperature for the vast majority, in spite of the fact that it relies upon your inclinations and propensities.

Test various temperatures to discover which is generally agreeable for you. Around 70°F (20°C) is best for a great many people.

11. Try not to Eat Late in the Evening

Late-evening eating may adversely affect both rest quality and the normal arrival of HGH and melatonin.

All things considered, the quality and sort of your late-night bite may assume a job also.

High-carb supper eaten four hours before bed helped individuals nod off faster Interestingly, one examination found that a low-carb diet likewise improved rest, showing that carbs are not constantly vital — particularly in the event that you are utilized to a low-carb diet.

Expending a huge dinner before bed can prompt poor rest and hormone interruption. In any case, certain dinners and snacks a couple of hours before bed may help.

12. Unwind and Clear Your Mind in the Evening

Numerous individuals have a pre-rest schedule that encourages them to unwind.

Unwinding procedures before bed have been appeared to improve rest quality and are another normal method used to treat a sleeping disorder.

A loosening up rub improved rest quality in individuals who were sick.

Methodologies incorporate tuning in to loosening up the music, perusing a book, scrubbing down, contemplating, profound breathing and representation.

Evaluate various strategies and find what works best for you.

Unwinding methods before bed, including hot showers and contemplation, may assist you with nodding off.

13. Wash up or Shower

A loosening up shower or shower is another well-known approach to rest better.

Studies demonstrate that they can improve in general rest quality and help individuals — particularly more established grown-ups — nod off faster.

A hot shower an hour and a half before bed improved rest quality and helped individuals get all the more profound rest.

Then again, on the off chance that you would prefer not to wash up around evening time, just washing your feet in boiling water can assist you with unwinding and improve rest.

A hot shower, shower or foot shower before bed can assist you with unwinding and improve your rest quality.

14. Preclude a Sleep Disorder

A hidden wellbeing condition might be the reason for your rest issues.

One basic issue is rest apnea, which causes conflicting and intruded on relaxing. Individuals with this issue quit breathing over and again while resting.

This condition might be more typical than you might suspect. One audit guaranteed that 24% of men and 9% of women have rest apnea.

Other basic medicinally analyzed issues incorporate rest development issue and circadian beat rest/wake issue, which are regular in move labourers.

In the event that you've generally battled with rest, it might be shrewd to counsel with your primary care physician.

There are numerous normal conditions that can cause poor rest, including rest apnea. See a specialist if poor rest is a reliable issue in your life.

15. Get a Comfortable Bed, Mattress and Pillow

A few people wonder why they generally rest better in an inn.
Aside from the loosening up condition, bed quality can likewise influence Sleep One investigation took a gander at the benefits of another bedding for 28 days, uncovering that it decreased back agony by 57%, shoulder torment by 60% and back solidness by 59%. It likewise improved rest quality by 60%.

Different examinations call attention to that new sheet material can improve rest. Furthermore, the low-quality sheet material can prompt expanded lower-back torment.

The best sleeping cushion and bedding is incredibly emotional. On the off chance that you are overhauling your bedding, base your decision on close to home inclination.

It is prescribed that you overhaul your bedding something like each 5–8 years.

On the off chance that you haven't swapped your sleeping pad or bedding for quite a long while, this can be fast — albeit perhaps costly — fix.

Your bed, bedding and pad can significantly affect rest quality and joint or back torment. Attempt to purchase a top-notch sleeping cushion and bedding each 5–8 years.

16. Exercise Regularly — But Not Before Bed

Exercise is extraordinary compared to other science-sponsored approaches to improve your rest and wellbeing.

It can upgrade all parts of rest and has been utilized to diminish the manifestations of a sleeping disorder.

One examination in more seasoned grown-ups verified that activity about split the measure of time it took to nod off and gave 41 additional minutes of rest around evening time.

In individuals with serious a sleeping disorder, the practice offered a larger number of benefits than most medications. Exercise decreased time to nod off by 55%, all-out night attentiveness by 30% and nervousness by 15% while expanding all-out rest time by 18%.

Albeit everyday practice is key for a decent night's rest, performing it past the point of no return in the day may mess rest up.

This is expected to the stimulatory impact of the activity, which expands readiness and hormones like epinephrine and adrenaline. Notwithstanding, a few investigations show no hindering effects, so it obviously relies upon the person.

Normal exercise during light hours is probably the ideal approaches to guarantee a decent night's rest.

17. Try not to Drink Any Liquids before Bed

Nighttime is the restorative term for over the top pee during the night. It influences rest quality and daytime vitality.

Drinking a lot of fluids before bed can prompt comparative indications; however, a few people are more delicate than others.

In spite of the fact that hydration is crucial for your wellbeing, it is insightful to diminish your liquid admission in the late night.

Make an effort not to drink any liquids 1–2 hours before heading to sleep.

You ought to likewise utilize the washroom directly before heading to sleep, as this may diminish your odds of waking in the night.

Decrease liquid admission in the late night and attempt to utilize the restroom directly before bed.

Rest assumes a key job in your wellbeing.

One huge survey connected deficient rest to an expanded heftiness danger of 89% in youngsters and 55% in grown-ups.

Different examinations reason that under 7–8 hours of the night expands your danger of creating coronary illness and type 2 diabetes.

On the off chance that you are keen on ideal wellbeing and prosperity, at that point you should focus on rest and fuse a portion of the tips above.

HEALTHY EXERCISES FOR WOMEN OVER 50 TP SUPPORT INTERMITTENT FASTING.

The beginning of the middle age is a basic point throughout everyday life. It is in the mid-50s when bulk starts to diminish, and fat stores start to develop. This can prompt heftiness, diabetes, hypertension, heart issues, stroke, and a few types of disease.

1. Try not to let your metabolism delayed down — do BURPEES.

High-power cardio invigorates our metabolism, which is more than would normally be appropriate to persuade after a specific age. So to forestall metabolism deceleration, we ought to do this activity on more than one occasion for each week. Start with one lot of 3 reps and include another redundancy each time. Try not to push yourself to an extreme.

2. Keep it firm — do SQUATS.

Each lady needs to have around backside; however, even the most fortunate ones who had it normally with no preparation will begin to lose it after the age of 40 gratitude to the decline of bulk. Appropriately done squats (with a straight back and knees directly above the feet) can condition your entire body and forestall damage by improving your adaptability.

3. To battle and forestall back torment — do a PLANK.

Doing this activity for 90 seconds 3 times each week is an extraordinary method to condition all the centre muscles of our bodies. It qualities our abs, the muscles of the chest, and the ones are encompassing the spine. Our whole waist fixes and bolsters our lower back.

4. Shield yourself from joint pain — push DUMBBELLS.

Incessant joint agony can assault grown-ups all things considered, so it's never too early to begin forestalling it, and perhaps the ideal approaches to do it is quality preparing. You don't need to go through hours lifting large weights. Doing deadlifts or overhead presses with 1-3 kg in each hand 2-3 times each week can do wonders for your body.

5. Allow your glutes to rest — do a GLUTE BRIDGE.

Sitting throughout the day in an office can deactivate our glutes which hinders the rate at which our body consumes calories — the metabolism. The hip expansion in the glute connect practice makes the butt work, and it can likewise open up any snugness from long periods of sitting. Leave your arms along your sides, press your butt muscles to lift your hips up, and crush them again at the top, at that point gradually drop your hips down.

6. Try not to let sarcopenia remove your muscles — do Y-TO-T RAISES.

Sarcopenia is a degenerative loss of skeletal muscle-related with ageing. So on the off chance that you'd prefer to forestall awful stance and back and shoulder hurts, it is imperative to reinforce the muscles of your back and shoulders.

7. Ensure your heart — train on an ELLIPTICAL MACHINE.

Low-sway cardio is an extraordinary route for women more than 40 to keep up a solid heart. In any case, on the off chance that you truly need your heart wellbeing to profit, you have to practice at 80% of your most extreme pulse for at any rate 30 minutes, 3 to 4 times each week. In the event that 10 is as hard as you can do on a size of one to 10, at that point you should work at the degree of 8.

8. Live effectively — WALK.

Strolling is the least difficult and the best exercise that anybody can do. While it consumes calories, conditions our body, and improves our mind-set, it additionally doesn't wear out our delicate joints, which is significant after a particular age.

9. Unwind — do YOGA.

Moderately aged women are increasingly inclined to get discouraged, as indicated by John Hopkins Medicine, one of the main social insurance frameworks in the United States. Yoga expands a disposition managing synapse, which is important to battle despondency. It likewise diminishes pressure and nervousness levels.

Do you know different exercises useful for women beyond 50 years old?

A complete exercise program ought to incorporate the accompanying:

1. Stretching expands bloodstream and prepares your body for work out. Extending additionally improves adaptability, facilitates development, and brings down the danger of damage and muscle strain. A warm-up and chill off time of 5 to 15 minutes ought to be done gradually and cautiously when a wide range of activity. Extending can help slacken muscles in the arms, shoulders, back, chest, stomach, hindquarters, thighs, and calves. It's additionally unwinding.

2. Aerobic exercise improves cardiovascular wellness and muscle tone. This sort of activity incorporates exercises, for example, strolling, running, swimming, cycling, moving, paddling, and cross country skiing.

3. Weight preparing (obstruction) practice advances muscle quality and adaptability.

Both high-impact and weight preparing activity can improve balance.

The 9 Exercise Tips

1. Wait at any rate of two hours in the wake of eating before energetic exercise.

2. Exercise just when feeling admirable.

3. Drink a lot of liquids both when working out.

4. Wear-free, open to attire that permits you to move effectively. Steady footwear intended for practice is an unquestionable requirement.

5. Set practical and safe objectives.

6. Avoid practising outside in exceptionally warm or freezing climate.

7. If you experience any of the accompanying side effects, quit practising promptly: chest torment or distress, unsteadiness, palpitations, or extreme brevity of breath.

8. Exercise with a companion.

9. Find an activity routine, teacher, as well as a program that you like, and have a great time!

RECIPES FOR BREAKFAST, LUNCH DINNER AND SNACKS.

BRAEKFAST RECIPES

What you truly need from your breakfast is excellent fuel brimming with supplements, micronutrients and phytonutrients that your body needs so as to get you during that time without glucose drops and with enough vitality to continue you.

So why not have a go at something new! I regularly start my day with a green smoothy. On the off chance that you like that though, read my blog 'Fledglings guide to smoothies' .on this website.

In any case, for somewhat more assortment, attempt a portion of my flavorful crude breakfast alternatives beneath. A crude 'grain-free' muesli, a natural product is serving of mixed greens with buckwheat and cashew yoghurt, a chia cacao pudding and a cinnamon banana porridge. Every one of these recipes is liberated from gluten and liberated from refined sugar. Give them a shot and let me know how you like them and how they affect you. Furthermore, recall, the key is assortment… don't simply eat something very similar consistently.

FATHEAD KETO CINNAMON ROLLS RECIPE - FAST and EASY

Everybody adores these keto cinnamon rolls! Just 40 minutes to make, with basic ingredients (no unique flour!), and they're delightful. For an astounding low carb dessert or keto breakfast, attempt this fathead cinnamon moves recipe.

Course Breakfast, Dessert

Cooking American

Calories 321 kcal

Planning Time 20 minutes

Cook Time 20 minutes

Absolute Time 40 minutes

Creator Maya Krampf from WholesomeYum.com

Servings cinnamon rolls

INGREDIENTS

- [ ]   2 cup Macadamia nuts (10 oz)

- [ ]   1/4 cup Erythritol

- [ ]   1 tbsp without gluten preparing powder

- [ ]   2 huge Egg

- [ ]   1 tsp Vanilla concentrate (discretionary)

- [ ]   4 cup Mozzarella cheddar (destroyed)

- [ ]   4 oz Cream cheddar

Filling

- [ ]   1/4 cup Butter (liquefied)

- [ ]   1/2 cup Erythritol

- [ ]   2 tbsp Cinnamon Icing

☐ 1/3 cup without sugar cream cheddar icing

☐ 1 tbsp unsweetened almond milk (or any milk of decision)

Directions

Spot the macadamia nuts into a food processor fitted with an S blade sharp edge. Heartbeat just until the nuts arrive at a fine, brittle consistency, without huge pieces. Try to beat, don't leave the food processor running, to attempt to make flour and not nut margarine. Scratch the sides varying. The nuts may, in any case, start to frame nut margarine a bit, yet attempt to maintain a strategic distance from however much as could reasonably be expected.

1.   Add the erythritol and preparing powder. Heartbeat two or multiple times, just until blended.

2.   Add the eggs and vanilla. Heartbeat two or multiple times once more, just until blended.

3.   Heat the mozzarella and cream cheddar in the microwave for around 2 minutes, mixing part of the way through and toward the end, or on the stove in a twofold heater, until simple to mix. Mix until smooth.

4.   Add the cheddar blend to the food processor. Push the cheddar blend down into the nut/egg blend. Heartbeat/puree until uniform batter structures, scratching down the sides vary. On the off chance that you experience difficulty getting it to blend, you can ply a little with a spatula and afterwards beat some more.

5.   Refrigerate the batter directly in the food processor for around 30-an hour, until the top is firm and not clingy.

6.   Meanwhile, preheat the broiler to 375 degrees F (191 degrees C). Line a 9x13 in (23x33 cm) heating skillet with material paper.

7.   Take the mixture out onto an enormous bit of material paper (not the one on the heating sheet). It will, at present, be genuinely clingy. Utilize a smidgen of the dissolved margarine on your hands to forestall staying as you spread it into a square shape. Spot another bit of material on top and turn out to a more slender square shape, around 14 in (36 cm) long X 10 in (25 cm) wide, and 1/3 X 1/2 in (8 to 13 mm) thick.

8.   Brush the mixture square shape with the greater part of the staying dissolved spread, leaving aside around 1-2 tablespoons. Mix together the erythritol and cinnamon for the filling. Sprinkle the blend uniformly over the square shape.

9.   Oil your hands again with the liquefied spread. Beginning from a long side of the square shape, fold up the batter into a log. As you come, oil the underside of the log as you strip it away from the material underneath during rolling. (This is to forestall breaking and staying.)

10.   Slice the sign into 1 in (2.5 cm) thick cuts, which will look like pinwheels. Spot the pinwheels level onto the lined heating dish, practically contacting yet not exactly.

11.   Bake for around 25 minutes, until the keto cinnamon rolls are brilliant on top. Cool for at any rate 20 minutes, until firm.

12.   Meanwhile, making the icing. Beat almond milk into the icing a tablespoon at once, until the icing is sufficiently meagre to sprinkle. When the keto cinnamon rolls are sufficiently firm, shower the icing over them.

NUTRITION INFORMATION PER SERVING

Nutrition Facts

Sum per serving. Serving size in recipe notes above.

Calories321

Fat29.5g

Protein11g

Complete Carbs5g

Net Carbs3g

Fiber2g

Sugar1g

Bacon, Spaghetti Squash Fritters Recipe

Planning Time

20 mins

Cook Time

20 mins

Complete Time

40 mins

It is ever considered how to cook spaghetti squash? Let me show the ideal way ever: Bacon Spaghetti Squash Fritters with Parmesan. These little spaghetti squash cakes are insane acceptable!

Course: Appetizer

Food: American

Servings: 8 misuses

Calories: 161 kcal

Ingredients

- 2 eggs

- 1/3 cup flour (for gluten free form, use multi-reason sans gluten King Arthur flour)

- 3 cups spaghetti squash, cooked and wrung out (see directions beneath)

- 1/2 cup Parmesan cheddar, newly ground

- 1/4 salt, in addition to extra, if necessary

- 3 green onions hacked

- 5 strips bacon, cooked, depleted of fat, and hacked

- 2 tablespoons olive oil

For embellish:

- 2 green onions hacked

- 1/4 cup Greek Yogurt

Directions

The most effective method to cook spaghetti squash:

1.   The recipe requires 3 CUPS COOKED spaghetti squash. 3 CUPS COOKED spaghetti squash is normally 1/2 or 2/3 of entire spaghetti squash. Initial 6 stages depict how to cook spaghetti squash in the stove (this should be possible at least 1 day ahead of time):

2.   Preheat stove to 425 Fahrenheit.

3.   Cut the squash in 2 parts, scratch out the seeds and the fibre out of every half. Splash oil over the cut sides of the squash. Shower the heating sheet with oil and spot the squash on the preparing sheet chop side down.

4.   Bake for around 30-40 minutes. Expel it from the stove when it's cooked through and delicate, and let it cool. Flip the squash so cut side faces up – that will accelerate the cooling after squash cools, scratch squash with a fork to evacuate substance in long strands and move to a bowl. Allow it to cool.

5.   Important: Wring out the simmered spaghetti squash by enveloping parts of it by paper towels and pressing hard with your hands over the sink. Be mindful so as not to drop the spaghetti squash into the sink if the paper towel breaks. Attempt to dispose of as a lot of fluid as you can.

6.   Roasted spaghetti squash can be refrigerated for 5 days. I like to cook spaghetti squash, refrigerate it and make wastes the following day or after 2 days - that permits spaghetti squash to deplete the fluid out and get dryer, which is ideal for squanders

Presently, on to how to make spaghetti squash squanders:

1.   In a huge bowl, utilizing an electric blender, beat 2 eggs on fast for 1-2 minutes. Include flour and keep beating for around 30 seconds to join. To a similar bowl, include spaghetti squash, Parmesan cheddar, 3 cleaved green onions, and 1/4 + 1/8 teaspoons salt. Blend very well until all the blend has a uniform consistency. Include cleaved bacon and blend. Taste and alter flavouring, if fundamental, despite the fact that it ought to be simply great.

2.   Heat an enormous skillet on high-medium warmth until VERY hot. At exactly that point include olive oil. It should sizzle and smoke immediately. Utilizing a tablespoon, spoon the

tablespoonful of the hitter for each misuse and drop on the skillet. Utilizing a spatula, right the state of each waste, making it compliment and rounder. Cook until the base side of each squander is brilliant dark coloured, around 1-2 minutes. Lessen warmth to medium. Utilizing a spatula, flip wastes to the contrary side, and cook 1-2 additional minutes. While flipping the squanders, you can utilize a spoon on the contrary side of the spatula to help push each misuse onto the spatula and afterwards flipping. Mood killer the warmth and let the squanders sit in the skillet (revealed) for 2-3 additional minutes (check the base to ensure it's not consumed - on the off chance that it is excessively dull, expel wastes from the skillet right away). Complete 4 misuses one after another, you ought to have an aggregate of 2 bunches (8 wastes all out).

3.   Serve as seems to be, or top with the dab of Greek yoghurt and hacked green onions (tasty whenever served thusly!).

Nutrition Facts

Bacon, Spaghetti Squash Fritters Recipe

Sum Per Serving (2 g)

Calories 161Calories from Fat 99

% Daily Value*

Fat 11g17%

Soaked Fat 3g19%

Cholesterol 54mg18%

Sodium 214mg9%

Potassium 112mg3%

Starches 7g2%

Sugar 1g1%

Protein 6g12%

Nutrient A 215IU4%

Nutrient C 2mg2%

Calcium 99mg10%

Iron 0.7mg4%

* Percent Daily Values depend on a 2000 calorie diet.

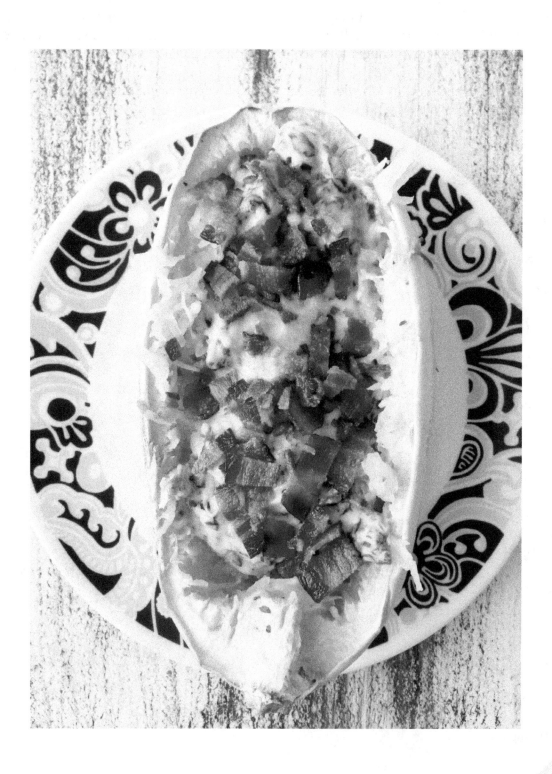

Keto Turmeric Milkshake

Keto turmeric milkshake is impeccable both hot and cold. The ideal sound beverage.

Prep Time5 mins

Absolute Time5 mins

Course: Breakfast, Drinks, Lunch, Snacks

Diet: Dairy Free, Gluten Free, Grain-free, Keto, LCHF, Low Carb, No Sugars, Paleo, Wheat Free

Catchphrase: Keto turmeric milkshake

Servings:

Absolute Carbs: 6.9g

Fibre: 1.4g

Ingredients

METRIC - CUPS/OUNCES

*   375 ml non-dairy milk I utilized coconut milk

*   2 tbsp coconut oil

*   3/4 tsp turmeric powder or 3 inches stripped turmeric root

*   1/2 tsp ginger powder or 1/2 inch stripped ginger root

*   1/4 tsp cinnamon

*   1/4 tsp vanilla

*   granulated sugar of decision or more, to your taste

*   pinch Himalayan salt

*   2 ice 3D shapes

Directions

1.   Place the entirety of the ingredients in a powerful blender. In the event that your blender isn't powerful enough, mesh or mince the turmeric and ginger roots before adding to the blender, or utilize powdered turmeric and ginger.

2.   Blend on HIGH for 30 seconds, or until thick and brilliant.

3.   Pout the kero turmeric milkshake into a glass and sprinkle with cinnamon and turmeric.

Notes

The nutrition board will fluctuate broadly relying upon which milk you choose to utilize, and it's fat substance.

Including ground dark pepper and fat may improve the assimilation of the dynamic compound in turmeric, curcumin. Make sure to consistently check with your human services proficient if turmeric will connect with your present drug or ailment.

Nutrition Facts

Keto Turmeric Milkshake

Sum Per Serving (1 serving)

Calories 351Calories from Fat 317

% Daily Value*

Fat 35.2g54%

Sugars 6.9g2%

Fibre 1.4g6%

Protein 1.6g3%

MATCHA GREEN TEA ENERGY BITES

- Prep Time: 2-5 minutes

- Total Time: 5 minutes

INGREDIENTS

- 1 cup destroyed coconut, unsweetened

- 4 Tbsp almond flour

- 2 Tbsp maple syrup, pretty much to taste*

- 1 Tbsp coconut oil

- 1 Tbsp matcha green tea

Guidelines

1. Blend everything together in a food processor.

2. Shape into 1″ balls and appreciate!

Store in the fridge.

LUNCH RECIPES

Your day by day work area lunch is looking miserable. Rather than agreeing to one more exhausting serving of mixed greens, stir up your late morning dinner routine with one of these insane delectable, soup, sandwich, and pasta recipes. Not exclusively will you top off on the great stuff (that implies no more post-lunch crash!), yet these simple-to-prepare recipes are truly moderate, which implies you'll have more cash to go through when the end of the week moves around. Obviously, smart dieting doesn't stop around early afternoon: Keep it going with one of these low-calorie dinners.

Triple Berry Salad with Candied Pecans

Planning Time

15 mins

Complete Time

15 mins

The BEST sweet lemon poppyseed dressing (no mayo), simply sweetened walnuts, and new berries over a bed of spinach. This berry spinach plate of mixed greens is flavorful and extraordinary to serve to a group!

Course: Salad

Cooking: American

Servings: 4 - 6 (as a side)

Creator: Chelsea

Ingredients

A plate of mixed greens

•   1 sack (6-8 ounces) new spinach OR plate of mixed greens mix (blended greens and spinach) ~7 cups

•   1 cup piling strawberries

•   1 cup piling raspberries

•   1 cup piling blackberries

- 4 ounces feta cheddar

Sweetened Pecans

- 1 enormous egg white

- 2 teaspoons water

- 1 teaspoon vanilla

- 1 cup white sugar

- 3/4 teaspoon salt

- 1 teaspoon cinnamon

- 4 cups walnut parts (1 pound)

Dressing

- 4 tablespoons crisply pressed lemon juice

- 1 teaspoon loading lemon get-up-and-go

- 1/4 teaspoon onion powder

- 1/2 teaspoon Dijon mustard doesn't utilize customary mustard

- 1/4 teaspoon salt

- 3 tablespoons white sugar

- 1/3 cup vegetable oil

- 1/2 tablespoon poppy seeds

Directions

A plate of mixed greens

1. Wash and THOROUGHLY dry (wet lettuce won't permit the dressing to follow well) the spinach. Expel any long stems.

2. Wash and altogether dry the organic product.

3.   Toss the natural product with the spinach. Include the sweetened walnuts and feta cheddar.

4.   Top with dressing just RIGHT before serving.

5.   If you plan on having scraps, don't hurl in with dressing as it doesn't store or sit well.

To treat the walnuts.

1.   Preheat broiler to 250 degrees F and liberally oil a preparing sheet.

2.   In a blending bowl, whip together the egg white, water, and vanilla until foamy. In a different bowl, combine sugar, salt, and cinnamon.

3.   Add walnuts to egg whites, mix to cover the nuts equitably. Expel the nuts, and hurl them in the sugar blend until covered. Spread the nuts out on the readied preparing sheet.

4.   Bake for 60 minutes, mixing and hurling at regular intervals.

Dressing:

1. Combine the naturally pressed lemon juice, lemon get-up-and-go, onion powder, dijon mustard, salt and sugar in a blender or food processor. Mix or heartbeat until totally smooth. Gradually pour in the vegetable oil and mix. Mix in the poppyseeds.

GLUTEN-FREE, LOW CARB and KETO FISH TACOS

Planning TIME: 20 MINUTES

COOK TIME: 15 MINUTES

MARINATING TIME: 2 HOURS

SERVINGS: TACOS

CALORIES: 48 KCAL

Preparing a clump of these gluten-free and keto fish tacos couldn't be simpler. The outcomes? An appropriately fresh outside, a flakey and delicate fish, and a general taste bomb of a low carb Mexican dish!

INGREDIENTS

FOR THE GLUTEN FREE and KETO FISH TACOS

- 250 g firm white-substance fish, for example, fumble or cod

- 1/3 cup acrid cream or coconut cream + 2 tsp apple juice vinegar

- 2 teaspoons apple juice vinegar

- 4 cloves garlic went through a press

- kosher salt to taste

- 1/2 cup whey protein disengage

- 1 teaspoon heating powder

- 1 1/2 teaspoon bean stew powder *see notes

- 1/4-1/2 teaspoon genuine salt to taste

- 1 egg

- 1 tablespoon harsh cream or coconut cream

- 2 teaspoons apple juice vinegar

- coconut oil or cooking oil of decision

SERVING SUGGESTIONS

- 1 cluster 15-minute keto and grain-free tortillas 8 tortillas

- 1 cluster pico de gallo salsa

- guacamole

- limes

METRIC - US Cups

Guidelines

1.   Mix harsh (or coconut) cream, vinegar, garlic and season to taste with salt. Cut the fish over the grain of the tissue into strips around 1/2 inch wide, and add it to the cream marinade. Cover and refrigerate for two hours, ideally medium-term.

2.   Make a cluster of our grain-free keto tortillas. You can have them moulded and all set for cooking them at the same time to the fish.

3.   Prepare your singing station by adding enough oil to a skillet or dish to make it around 1/2-inch down. You can spare a great deal of oil by utilizing a smaller dish and broiling in groups. Warmth up oil over medium/low warmth while you coat the fish.

4.   Mix the whey protein, preparing powder, bean stew powder and salt in a shallow plate or dish. In a subsequent plate or dish, whisk the egg with cream and vinegar.

5.   Coat the fish by delicately expelling overabundance marinade, plunging in the egg blend, trailed by the whey protein blend, promptly setting in the hot oil and treating the upper immediately. You need to broil the fish directly in the wake of covering for best freshness. Fry on the two sides until profound brilliant and move to a paper-lined plate for two or three minutes.

6.   Serve immediately with the newly made tortillas, a lot of limes and your salsa of decision.

RECIPE NOTES

Or prepare your own stew powder blend: 3/4 tsp paprika, 1/4 tsp garlic powder, 1/4 tsp onion powder, 1/4 tsp dried oregano, 1/8 tsp cayenne pepper, 1/8 tsp dried cumin.
It will be ideal if you note that nutrition realities were assessed for the fish just, include 2g net carbs per keto tortilla. Likewise, remember that evaluating a totally exact examination for these is essentially unthinkable given the marinade, searing oil and so on. Having said that, the fish and covering itself is essentially carb-less.

Nutrition Facts

Gluten-Free, Low Carb and Keto Fish Tacos

Sum Per Serving (1 fish taco)

Calories 48

% Daily Value*

Cholesterol 33mg11%

Sodium 104mg4%

Potassium 194mg6%

Protein 9g18%

Nutrient A 155IU3%

Nutrient C 0.3mg0%

Calcium 30mg3%

Iron 0.3mg2%

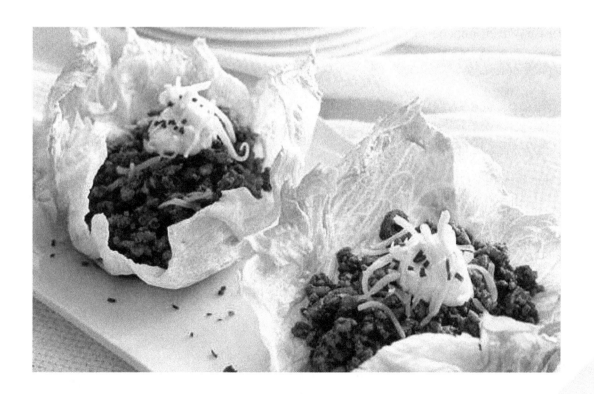

Fast and EASY CHICKEN SPRING ROLL JARS

These Fast and Easy Chicken Spring Roll Jars are the ideal get and go lunch. Amass the noodles, ground chicken and veggies early and include a little sweet bean stew sauce for some kick!

4.5 from 10 votes

Planning Time: 15 minutes

Cook Time: 15 minutes

All out Time: 30 minutes

Servings: 4 containers

Calories: 480kcal

INGREDIENTS

- 1 tbsp sesame oil

- 1 lb ground chicken or turkey

- 2 tbsp soy sauce

- 2 cloves garlic minced

- 1 tbsp ginger, minced

- 1 pack coleslaw

- 2 tsp soy sauce

- 1/2 cup sweet bean stew sauce

- 1 cup cucumber, cut into matchsticks

- 1 cup red pepper, cut

- 2 cups cooked vermicelli noodles

- 1/3 cup cilantro, slashed (can likewise utilize/include new mint and basil)

- Sesame seeds, soy sauce and sriracha to taste

Guidelines

1.   Heat sesame oil over prescription high warmth in a huge skillet. Include ground chicken and 2 tbsp soy sauce, cooking for 2-3 min. Include garlic and ginger, at that point sautee for 7-8 min until chicken is completely cooked.

2.   Remove chicken from skillet and include coleslaw and 2 tsp soy sauce, sauteing for 2-3 min until slaw is somewhat shrivelled. In the meantime, cook vermicelli noodles as indicated by bundle bearings (typically takes 2-3 min in bubbling water).

3.   Divide sweet bean stew sauce among the base of 4 medium-sized artisan containers (it winds up being around 2 tbsp sweet bean stew sauce added to each 16oz container). Gap chicken among containers, at that point coleslaw, cucumber and red pepper. Top with vermicelli noodles, crisp herbs and sesame seeds. Include soy sauce and sriracha whenever wanted. Containers keep in ice chest as long as 5 days.

NUTRITION

Calories: 480kcal | Carbohydrates: 73g | Protein: 32g | Fat: 7g | Saturated Fat: 1g | Cholesterol: 62mg | Sodium: 1172mg | Potassium: 686mg | Fiber: 5g | Sugar: 21g | Vitamin A: 1329IU | Vitamin C: 90mg | Calcium: 66mg | Iron: 2mg

SMOKEY GREEN BEAN TURKEY SKILLET

- Prep Time: 5 minutes

- Cook Time: 15 minutes

- Total Time: 20 minutes

- Yield: 4 servings 1x

Portrayal

At last, a ground turkey recipe that has nothing to do with tacos! This Smokey Green Bean Turkey Skillet has an astounding smokey season yet is adaptable enough to partition over rice, quinoa or pasta. Ideal for feast preparing!

INGREDIENTS

- 1 tablespoon olive oil (or avo oil)

- 1 pound lean ground turkey

- 1/2 teaspoon garlic, minced

- 1 red chile pepper, diced

- 1/2 yellow onion, diced

- 2 cups new green beans, closes expelled, cut into 1 or 2-inch lengths (around 8 oz)

- 2 teaspoons smoke flavouring mix (see note for choices)

- 3/4 cup chipotle salsa (any salsa will work)

- pinch of salt

- optional: present with rice, quinoa, pasta, greens

Directions

1.   Heat olive oil in a huge skillet over medium-high warmth. Include ground turkey and break separated with a spatula. Include a spot of salt. Cook until meat is almost cooked through, around 4-5 minutes. Expel overabundance fluid from skillet.

2.   Push turkey meat to the other side of the skillet. Include red pepper, onion, green beans, and garlic. Combine meat and vegetables and saute for 3-4 additional minutes, mixing once in a while.

3.   Add flavouring and salsa. Blend ingredients in the skillet until uniformly disseminated. Decrease warmth to low, and stew for 6-7 minutes or until green beans are delicate, mixing sporadically.

4.   Serve over rice, quinoa, or pasta! Store in an impermeable holder in the cooler for as long as 4 days.

NUTRITION

• Serving Size: 1/4 of dish

• Calories: 312

• Fat: 15.6g

• Carbohydrates: 8g

• Protein: 34.9g

SLOW COOKER CARNITAS BURRITO BOWLS

Remove an hour from your day to prepare these astounding moderate cooker carnitas burrito bowls! We'll tell you the best way to make Crockpot carnitas and even toss in headings for Instant Pot carnitas so you can make the most epic dinner prep burrito bowls around town!

- PREP TIME:20 minutes

- COOK TIME:6 hours

- TOTAL TIME:6 hours 20 minutes

YIELD: 4 1x

Class: Dinner

Strategy: Slow Cooker

Cooking: Mexican

INGREDIENTS

PORK CARNITAS

- 1 pound pork midsection or pork butt (choice to utilize chicken bosom)

- 3 tablespoons olive oil, partitioned

- 1 tablespoon minced garlic

- 1 tablespoons squeezed orange

- 1/3 cup lime juice

- 3 teaspoons ground cumin

- 2 teaspoons smoked paprika

- salt and pepper, to taste

- 4 oz. can green chiles

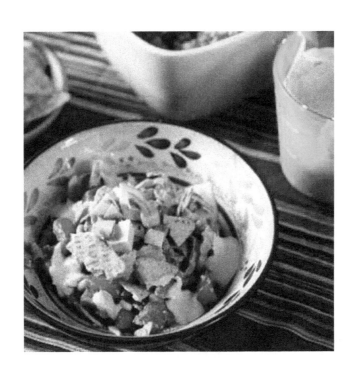

- 1 15-oz. can yellow sweet corn, depleted

- 2 tablespoons lime juice

- 1/2 tablespoon apple juice vinegar

- 2 tablespoons slashed cilantro, new

- 1/3 cup red onion, finely slashed

- 1/3 cup cotija cheddar, disintegrated

- 1/2 teaspoon paprika

- salt and pepper, to taste

CILANTRO LIME BROWN RICE

Different INGREDIENTS

- 1 15-oz. can dark beans

- 4–8 cups romaine lettuce

- Lime wedges

Directions

PORK CARNITAS

1.   Place around 2 tablespoons of olive on the base of a huge dish. Warmth to medium/high warmth. Burn pork on all sides for 1 moment for each side.

2.   Transfer singed pork into your moderate cooker and include somewhat more olive oil and garlic. Go warmth to low and cook for 6-8 hours*.

3.   Once the pork is delicate, expel pork and shred with 2 forks. Spot destroyed pork and around 1/4 cup – 1/3 cup of the juice from the moderate cooker into a huge bowl and include the remainder of the carnitas ingredients and blend.

ROAD CORN SALAD

1.   Place all ingredients into a medium-size bowl and blend.

CILANTRO LIME BROWN RICE

BOWL ASSEMBLY

1.   Place around 2 cups of romaine lettuce on the base of your bowl. At that point include 1/4 of the meat (4 oz.), around 3/4 cup cilantro lime darker rice, 1/2 cup road corn, and 1/4 cup dark beans.

2.   Serve with crisp lime and more cotija!

NOTES

•   Slow Cooker: We prescribe cooking for 6-8 hours on low for delicate pork, be that as it may, in the event that you are in a surge, you can cook the pork on high for 2-4 hours.

•   Instant Pot: If you'd prefer to make Instant Pot Carnitas, turn your Instant Pot to the saute capacity. Add olive oil to the base and burn all sides of your pork for 1 moment. At that point, turn your Instant Pot off and include garlic and somewhat more olive oil to your Instant Pot. Close cover, turn the valve to seal and cook on manual high for 60 to an hour and a half when the clock has gone off, fast discharge your Instant Pot to let out the steam. Shred and include the remainder of the carnitas ingredients. An alternative to follow THIS recipe.

NUTRITION

•   Serving Size: 1/4

•   Calories: 407

•   Sugar: 5

•   Fat: 18

•   Carbohydrates: 29

•   Fibre: 12

•   Protein: 32

CUMIN SPICED BEEF WRAPS – LOW CARB, PALEO

•   Prep Time: 15 minutes

- Cook Time: 10 minutes

- Total Time: 25 minutes

- Yield: Makes 2 Servings 1x

INGREDIENTS

- 1–2 tbsp coconut oil

- 1/4 onion, diced little

- 2/3 lb ground meat

- 1 red chile pepper, diced little

- 2 tbsp cilantro, hacked

- 1 tsp ginger, minced

- 4 cloves garlic, minced

- 2 tsp cumin

- Salt and pepper, to taste

- 8 huge cabbage leaves (savoy cabbage or Napa cabbage)

Directions

1.   Place 1-2 tbsp of coconut oil into a skillet and sauté the onions, ground hamburger, and peppers on medium warmth.

2.   When the ground meat is cooked, include the cilantro, ginger, garlic, cumin, salt, and pepper to taste.

3.   Fill a huge pot 3/4 full with water and heat to the point of boiling.

4.   Using tongs, whiten each cabbage leaf in the bubbling water (put each leaf into the bubbling water for 20 seconds). At that point dive each leaf into some virus water before depleting and putting onto a plate.

5.   Spoon the meat blend onto every lettuce leaf and overlay into a roll.

Nutritional facts

Per Serving – Calories: 375, Fat: 26g | Protein: 30g, Total Carbs: 6g | Fiber: 2g | Net Carbs: 4g

INTERMITTENT FOR DINNER RECIPES

Chicken and Broccoli Stir Fry

This recipe for chicken and broccoli pan-fried food is an exemplary dish of chicken sauteed with crisp broccoli florets and covered in an appetizing sauce. You can have a solid and simple dinner on the table in under 30 minutes!

CourseMain

CuisineAsian

Keywordbroccoli sautéed food, chicken and broccoli pan sear, chicken pan-fried food.

Prep Time10 minutes

Cook Time20 minutes

All out Time30 minutes

Servings

Calories308kcal

INGREDIENTS

- 1 pound boneless skinless chicken bosom cut into 1 inch pieces

- 1 tablespoon + 1 teaspoon vegetable oil

- 2 cups little broccoli florets

- 1 cup cut mushrooms on the off chance that you don't care for mushrooms you can include more broccoli

- 2 teaspoons minced crisp ginger

- 1 teaspoon minced garlic

- 1/4 cup clam sauce

- 1/4 cup low sodium chicken broth or water

- 1 teaspoon sugar

- 2 teaspoons toasted sesame oil

- 1 teaspoon soy sauce

- 1 teaspoon cornstarch

- salt and pepper to taste

Guidelines

1. Heat 1 teaspoon of oil in an enormous skillet over medium warmth. Include the broccoli and mushrooms and cook for around 4 minutes or until vegetables are delicate.

2. Add the ginger and garlic to the skillet and cook for 30 seconds more.

3. Remove the vegetables from the skillet; place them on a plate and spread.

4. Wipe the skillet clean with a paper towel and turn the warmth to high. Include the rest of the tablespoon of oil.

5. Season the chicken pieces with salt and pepper and add them to the container in a solitary layer - you may need to do this progression in clusters. Cook for 3-4 minutes on each side until brilliant darker and cooked through.

6. Add the vegetables back to the skillet and cook for 2 additional minutes or until the vegetables are warmed through.

7. In a bowl whisk together the clam sauce, chicken broth, sugar, sesame oil and soy sauce. In a little bowl blend the cornstarch in with a tablespoon of cold water.

8.   Pour the shellfish sauce blend over the chicken and vegetables; cook for 30 seconds. Add the cornstarch and heat to the point of boiling; cook for 1 progressively minute or until the sauce has quite recently begun to thicken.

9.   Serve fastly, with rice whenever wanted.

NUTRITION

Calories: 308kcal | Carbohydrates: 15g Protein: 37g | Fat: 12g | Saturated Fat: 2g | Cholesterol: 96mg | Sodium: 796mg | Fiber: 1g | Sugar: 6g

MISO SOUP RECIPE

Planning TIME 10 MINUTES

COOK TIME 20 MINUTES

All out TIME 30 MINUTES

Supporting miso soup with ginger, garlic, vegetables and tofu is a superb one-pot feast.

INGREDIENTS

- 2 tablespoons additional virgin olive oil

- 1 yellow onion, stripped and diced

- 1 tablespoon stripped new ground ginger, in addition to additional for serving

- 4 cloves garlic, minced

- 2 celery stalks, daintily cut

- 2 carrots, hacked or spiralized

- 1 Japanese sweet potato, hacked or spiralized (or 1 zucchini)

- 6 cups of water

- 5 tablespoons white miso glue

- 1 cup shelled edamame

- 7 oz. additional firm natural tofu, depleted and cubed

- 4 huge stalks kale, stem expelled and daintily cut

- ocean salt to taste

- 1 cup bean grows

- 3 green onions, daintily cut

Directions

1. Add the oil to a huge pot set over medium warmth. Include the onion and saute until mollified, around 5 minutes. Include the ginger and garlic and saute one more

moment. Include the celery, carrot, and sweet potato if utilizing. Saute two minutes. Add the water and bring to a stew. Stew until veggies start to mollify.

2.   Carefully exchange one cup of the warm water a bowl and rush in the miso glue. This will enable the glue to blend into the water all the more effectively. Empty the miso water into the pot and mix to join. Delicately stew until vegetables are cooked through. Include edamame, tofu, and cut kale and stew until kale has shrivelled, around one moment. Expel from heat. Add salt to taste. Top with bean sprouts and green onions. I like to grind a squeeze all the more crisp ginger over the highest point of my soup. However that is discretionary.

Nutrition Information:

Sum Per Serving: CALORIES: 269 TOTAL FAT: 12g SATURATED FAT: 2g TRANS FAT: 0g UNSATURATED FAT: 10g CHOLESTEROL: 0mg SODIUM: 1036mg CARBOHYDRATES: 30g FIBER: 8g SUGAR: 9g PROTEIN: 15g

Darkened Salmon with Avocado Salsa

Salmon prepared with a scrumptious cajun flavour mix and seared until firm served bested with cool and velvety avocado salsa!

Today I have a too speedy, simple and delectable supper for you, a darkened salmon with avocado salsa. This recipe couldn't be more straightforward, you simply season the salmon with a cajun flavouring and afterwards sear it until fresh and serve it beat with cool and velvety avocado salsa. The cajun flavouring is loaded with the season and incorporates a hot warmth that goes consummately with the rich salmon and the crisp avocado salsa. The salmon is sautéed at high warmth in a skillet until the skin and outside are decent and firm and the inside stays pleasant and sodden and delicate. The avocado salsa goes incredibly well with the darkened salmon where the fresh and succulent cucumber adds a stunning surface to everything. This darkened salmon with avocado salsa is the ideal speedy, light and delicious feast to commence the New Year!

The avocado and cucumber salsa!

Darkened Salmon with Avocado Salsa

Prep Time:5 minutes Cook Time:10 minutes Total Time:15 min.

The Servings: 4

Salmon prepared with a delicious cajun flavour mix and seared until fresh served bested with cool and velvety avocado salsa!

ingredients

For the darkened salmon:

- 1 tablespoon oil

- 4 (6 ounces) pieces salmon

- 4 teaspoons cajun flavouring

For the avocado salsa:

- 2 avocado, diced

- 1/4 cup red onion, diced

- 1 jalapeno, finely diced

- 1 tablespoon cilantro, hacked

- 1 tablespoon lime juice

- salt to taste

For the avocado and cucumber salsa:

- 2 avocado, diced

- 1 cup cucumber, diced

- 1/4 cup green onion, diced

- 1 tablespoon parsley, hacked

- 1 tablespoon lemon juice

- salt to taste

bearings

For the darkened salmon:

1. Heat the oil in an overwhelming base skillet over medium-high warmth, including the salmon, prepared with the cajun flavouring, and cook until profoundly brilliant dark coloured to somewhat darkened before flipping and rehashing for the opposite side.

1. For the avocado salsa:

2. Mix everything and appreciate on the salmon!

3. For the avocado and cucumber salsa:

4. Mix everything and appreciate on the salmon!

Alternative: Use trout, tilapia or other fish rather than salmon.

The Nutritional Facts: Calories 445, Fat 31.5g (Saturated 5.8g, Trans 0), Cholesterol 76mg, Sodium 72mg, Carbs 9.9g (Fiber 7.1g, Sugars 1.0g), Protein 35.1g

Buttered Cod in Skillet

An astounding, speedy and simple recipe for buttered cod in skillet. Prepared shortly, this fish recipe has a wow factor. The prepared cod cooked in the spread and bested with herbs and lemon juice is stunning.

Prep Time5 mins

Cook Time5 mins

All out Time10 mins

Course: Dinner

Food: American

Watchword: buttered cod, cod recipe

Servings: 4 servings

Calories: 294kcal

Creator: Valentina's Corner

Ingredients

Cod-

☐   1 1/2 lbs cod filets

☐   6 Tbsp unsalted margarine, cut

Flavouring

☐   ¼ tsp garlic powder

☐   ½ tsp table salt

☐   ¼ tsp ground pepper

☐   ¾ tsp ground paprika

☐   Few lemon cuts

☐   Herbs, parsley or cilantro

Guidelines

Step by step instructions to Make Buttered Cod in Skillet-

Stir together ingredients for flavouring in a little bowl.

1. Cut cod into littler pieces, whenever wanted. Season all sides of the cod with the flavouring.

2. Heat 2 Tbsp margarine in a huge skillet over medium-high warmth. When margarine softens, add cod to skillet. Cook 2 minutes.

3. Turn warmth down to medium. Turn cod finished, top with outstanding margarine and cooked another 3-4 minutes.

4. Butter will totally dissolve, and the fish will cook. (Try not to overcook the cod, it will get soft and totally self-destruct.)

5. Drizzle cod with crisp lemon juice. Top with crisp herbs, whenever wanted. Serve right away.

Nutrition Facts

Buttered Cod in Skillet

Sum Per Serving

Calories 294Calories from Fat 162

% Daily Value*

Fat 18g28%

Immersed Fat 11g69%

Cholesterol 118mg39%

Sodium 385mg17%

Potassium 712mg20%

Protein 30g60%

Nutrient A 815IU16%

Nutrient C 1.7mg2%

Calcium 32mg3%

Iron 0.7mg4%

Cooked Lemon Butter Garlic Shrimp and Asparagus

ONE PAN Roasted Lemon Garlic Butter Shrimp and Asparagus hurled with bean stew chips, and new parsley isn't just overflowing with season however on your table in 15 MINUTES! No joke! This recipe is the simplest, most fulfilling supper that preferences absolutely gourmet. Load up on solidified shrimp, and you can make this rich-tasting dinner at minute's notification. Serve the (adjustable warmth) fiery lemon garlic spread shrimp plain or transform it into lemon garlic margarine shrimp pasta!

Prep Time   10 minutes

Cook Time   12 minutes

Servings   - 6 servings

INGREDIENTS

Asparagus

- 1 pound dainty/medium asparagus closes cut

- 1 tablespoon olive oil

- 1 garlic clove, minced

- 1/4 teaspoon salt

- 1/8 teaspoon pepper Shrimp

- 1 1/2 pounds medium uncooked stripped shrimp deveined*

- 1 tablespoon olive oil

- 2-3 garlic cloves, minced

- 1/2 teaspoon salt

- 1/4 teaspoon paprika

- 1/8 teaspoon pepper

- 1/8-1/4 teaspoon red pepper chips

- 3 tablespoons slashed new parsley

- 1 1/2 tablespoons lemon juice or more to taste

- 3 tablespoons margarine, cubed

Present with

- Pasta

- Rice

Guidelines

1. Preheat broiler to 400 degrees F.

2. Line a Jelly Roll Pan (10x15) with thwart and gently splash with cooking shower. Include asparagus and shower with 1 tablespoon olive oil. Include 1 minced garlic clove, 1/4 teaspoon salt and 1/8 teaspoon pepper. Hurl until uniformly covered at that point line asparagus in a solitary layer. Cook for 4-6 minutes relying upon thickness.

3. Meanwhile, expel tails from shrimp.

4. Remove container from the stove and push asparagus to the other side of the dish (keep in a solitary layer). Include shrimp and sprinkle with 1 tablespoon olive oil. Include 2-3 minced garlic cloves (or more to taste), 1/2 teaspoonful of salt, 1/4 teaspoonful of paprika, 1/8 teaspoon pepper, 1/8-1/4 teaspoon red bean stew pieces and crisp parsley. Hurl until equally covered at that point line shrimp in a solitary layer.

5. Top asparagus with 1 tablespoon cubed spread, uniformly divided. Top shrimp with 2 tablespoons cubed margarine, uniformly separated. Broil for 6 minutes or just until shrimp is murky.

6. Remove dish from stove and shower with lemon juice. Season with extra salt and pepper to taste. Present with pasta, rice, and so forth.

RECIPE NOTES

*Weigh your 11/2 pounds shrimp with tails on, at that point expel tails. In the event that buys shrimp with the tails previously evacuated, alter weight in like manner.

CPSIA information can be obtained
at www.ICGtesting.com
Printed in the USA
LVHW060750260421
685569LV00010B/527